Ease into Yoga for Men and Women

A path to better life: better health, longer life and, yes, better sex

1st Edition

by
50 year old Yogi

Contents

Introduction

The Book

The idea behind this book is different then many other Yoga books. It is meant to introduce you to Yoga through the long term (minimum 12 months) step by step program. The book is divided into several sections or phases. You will progress from one section to the next.

While this book contains everything you need to follow the program all by yourself you should consider joining us online as well.

Yoga Program

This Yoga program was created with men in mind, especially those over 40. However, the poses presented here can be performed by men and women of any age and at any level of fitness. They are straightforward yet highly beneficial.

The Yoga poses selected for this book warm up the body and tone your muscles. They are excellent for practically EVERYONE because they stretch and strengthen all the major muscle groups. Some of the poses/exercises have been also used in martial arts and other sports. In a short period of time, you will feel healthier and in much better shape. You will also enjoy an improved sex life. Your performance will improve on many different levels.

This Yoga program is just the exercises, no religious or spiritual elements. So, no OMs and other chants. For example: one of the routines is called "Sun Salutations", but please be assured it's just a name and not a sun worshiping ceremony.

Men's Yoga

While the latest trends made Yoga look like an activity for women, it simply is not true. Men can benefit from Yoga as much as women do. While, in the West, the women are the driving force of popularity of yoga we have to recognize that men have always practiced yoga. Only recently it became more popular among women than men. Possibly, because in the modern times men are more inclined to do the competitive sports and there is no competition in yoga. Also, men can feel uneasy in the yoga class when women are more flexible and can do most poses without much effort.

You may think that yoga is just stretching, But it is more than that. Yoga is about developing both strength and flexibility. The poses shown here can be done quickly, to warm-up your body, or slowly to increase stamina and perfection of the pose.

I will also introduce exercises other then yoga. They will be just as easy to perform and are very beneficial to your health. They will be separate because they are performed more like Pilates then Yoga.

The most noteworthy thing about this program is that you will stop feeling intimidated by Yoga.

I want you to try and do it, and I want you to have fun doing it! Every few days take a break from Yoga and do something else. After you are done with the program take one or two Yoga classes. Compare what you do with what others are doing. Treat your Yoga workout as part of your life style. You will be surprised how enjoyable it feels.

Benefits of Yoga

Yoga teaches you how to move your body in new ways. It offers the immense health benefits by enabling you to develop your balance, strength, and flexibility.

Benefit #1: Flexibility
When people, especially men, think of yoga, they see pictures of women stretching like gymnasts and they imagine having to do that too. That makes them worry that they're too old, inflexible or unfit to do yoga. However, the truth is you're never too old to improve any of those.

The yoga poses work by stretching your muscles and soft tissues. This loosens tight muscles and increases the range of motion in joints. The outcome is a sense of fluidity and inner strength throughout your body.

Benefit #2: Healthy Heart
Yoga has been known to lower blood pressure and slower the heart rate. A slower heart rate can benefit people with heart disease and in danger of stroke. Yoga has also been associated with decreased cholesterol levels as well as a boost in immune system.

Benefit #3: Better Posture
With increased flexibility, and strength comes a better posture. Most standing and sitting yoga poses develop core strength. With a stronger core, you're more likely to sit and stand "tall."

Benefit #4: Better Breathing
Because of the deep breathing used in yoga, lung capacity often improves. With improved lung capacity comes better sports performance and endurance.

Benefit #5: Less Stress
Even beginners tend to feel less stressed and more relaxed after their first yoga session. Yoga meditation techniques calm your mind or quiet the "mind chatter" often associated with stress. So, the more you do yoga the less stressed you will be.

Benefit #6: Strength
Practicing yoga will help you improve muscle tone. Many of the poses, such as Downward Dog (found in Sun Salutations), Upward Dog, Cobra, and Plank pose (Sun Salutations), build upper-body strength. The standing poses build strength in your hamstrings, quadriceps, and abdominal

muscles. This becomes crucial as people age.

Benefit #7: Concentration and mood
Harder to pin down and research scientifically, concentration and the ability to focus mentally are common benefits mentioned by yoga students. The same is true with mood.

Benefit #8: Improved Sex Life
Yoga is a true physical and mental workout, so it's no surprise it can help you have better sex. Yoga promotes sexual vitality, treats premature ejaculation and enhances women's libido.

Warnings:
- Pregnant women should not practice after the third month of pregnancy
- Anybody with high blood pressure is warned against some postures (shoulder stand and the plow).
- People with recent or chronic injury to the back, knees or hips, should consult their physicians.
- If you have any doubts or concerns, please consult your physician about Yoga practice.

Before we start

What you need the most is a simple yoga mat. There are products out there claiming to be both Yoga and Pilates' mats. **Please ignore them!** Yoga mats need to be thin. You have to be able to feel the floor. They also have to be "sticky" to prevent slipping. Pilates mats are thicker, often twice as thick as yoga mats, because the floor exercises (in Pilates it's about 90% of all exercises) usually require additional padding. Also, unlike in Yoga, in Pilates there is no requirement to "feel the floor". Extra thick yoga mats may pose a problem when performing balance poses.

Yoga mats can be found in stores like Walmart, Marshalls and Target priced from $13.00 to $30.00.

The second item(s) you need is a pair of sweat pants. They need to be loose, warm and comfortable not necessary the "yoga pants".

Phase 1

This phase will last only 1 week. Please workout 3 days a week. For example: Monday, Wednesday and Friday or Tuesday, Thursday and Saturday.

We will start with breathing:
- Sit on the mat in a neutral posture and place your hands on the knees.
- Relax your shoulders.
- Slowly deeply inhale (as you would in your doctors office). Hold for 2 seconds.
- Exhale.
- Repeat for a total of 10 deep breaths.

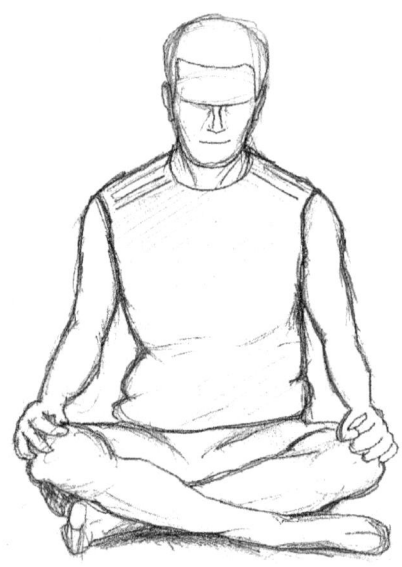

Fig. 1: Neutral Posture

Neck stretching:
- Turn your head up. Look up at the ceiling.
- Turn your head down, "Chin to Chest", look down.
- Repeat, turn your head up.
- Turn your head down.
- Look straight ahead.
- Turn your head 90 degrees to the left.
- Turn back to look straight ahead.
- Turn your head 90 degrees to the right.

- Repeat, turn your head to the left.
- Turn back to look straight ahead.
- Turn your head to the right.
- Look straight ahead.
- Clockwise head rotation – twice.
- Counterclockwise head rotation – twice.

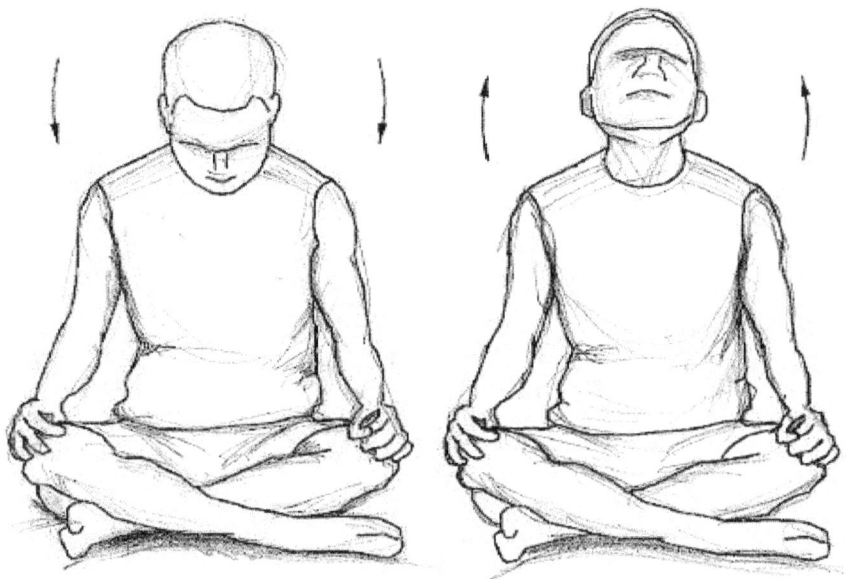

Fig. 2: Head up & down

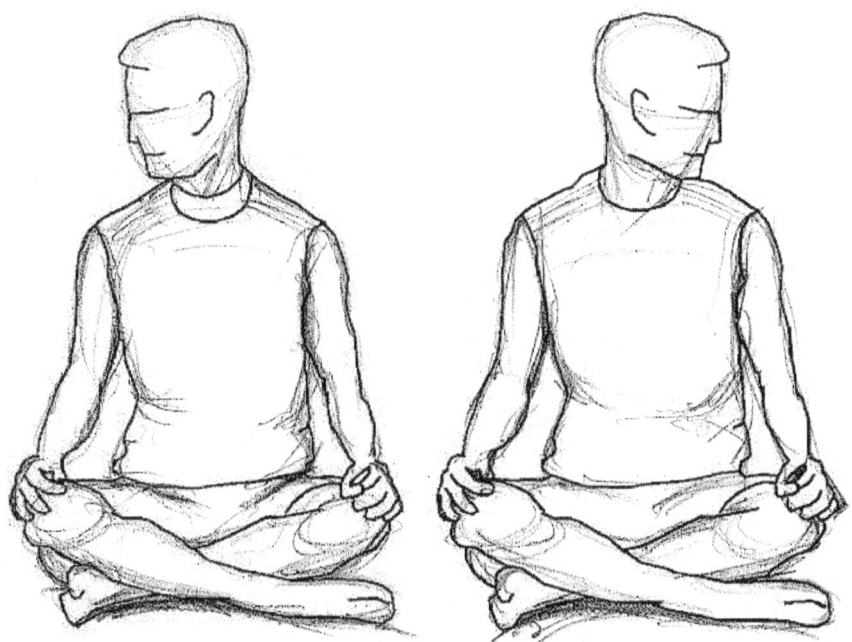

Fig. 3: Head left & right

Shoulders:

- Shrug your shoulders: while your palms are resting on your knees lift your shoulders and hold for 2 seconds. Let your shoulders drop. Rest for 2 seconds and repeat the shrugs two more times.
- Touch your left ear with your right hand.
- Place your left hand under the elbow of your right hand. Apply pressure on the elbow to force the right hand go farther behind your left ear.
- Repeat on the other side.

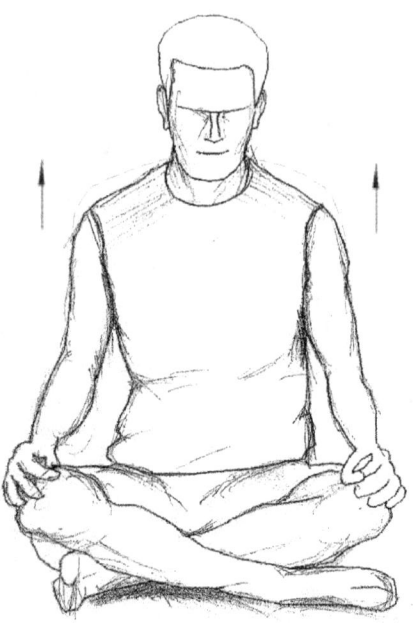

Fig. 4: Shoulder Shrug

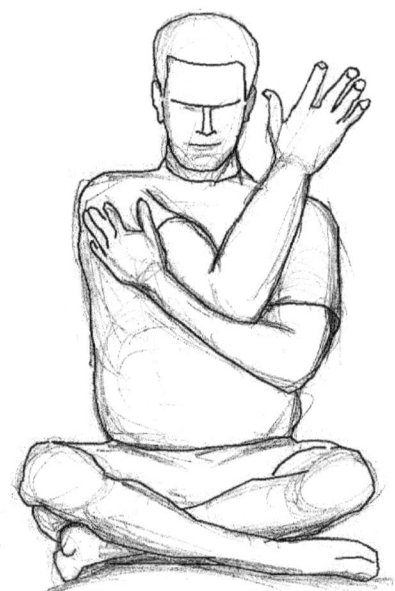

Fig. 5: Shoulder Stretch

Bow (toe touches):
- Stand with the feet close together
- Bring your palms together and raise to the chest level as if you were praying.
- Raise your clasped arms over your head trying to stretch your body upward.
- Now, bow and touch your toes.
- Hold for 2 seconds.
- Straighten up bringing your arms up to your chest.
- Repeat one more time.

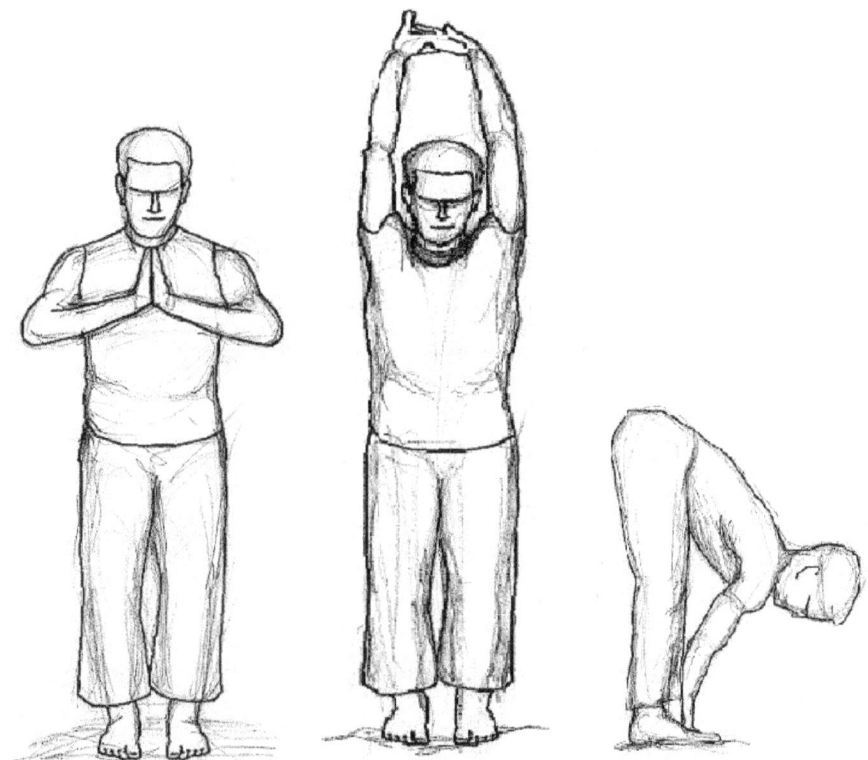

Fig. 6: Toe touches

Plank Pose / Cobra Pose:
- Stand with feet together, arms at your sides.
- Step back to push-up position (Plank Pose).
- Lower your body to the floor (belly, chest & legs should touch the floor).
- Raise your upper body by pushing out with your hands (Cobra Pose). Hold 5 seconds.
- Lower your body to the floor.

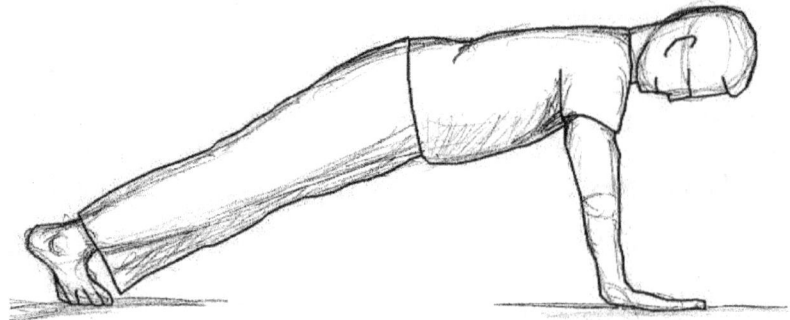

Fig. 7: Plank Pose

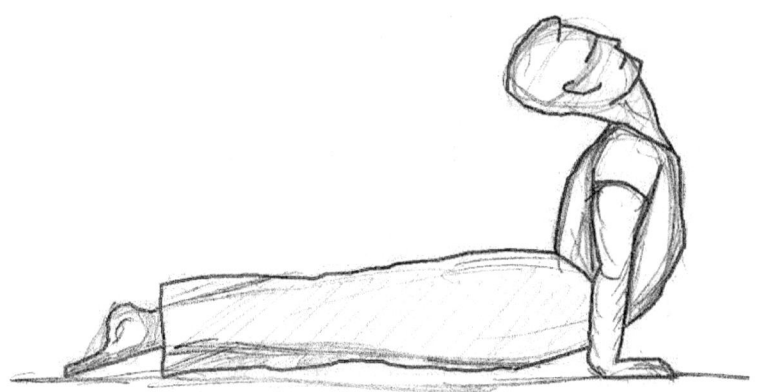

Fig. 8: Cobra Pose

Head to the Knee:
- Sit with straight legs in front of you.
- Pull the left leg to the center and place the foot sole lightly against the inner thigh of the right leg so the shin is at a right angle to the right leg.
- While holding the left ankle (with the left hand) grab the right ankle with the other hand. Pull your head to the right knee.
- This is the Head to Knee Pose. Stay in it for 5 seconds.
- Repeat on other side.

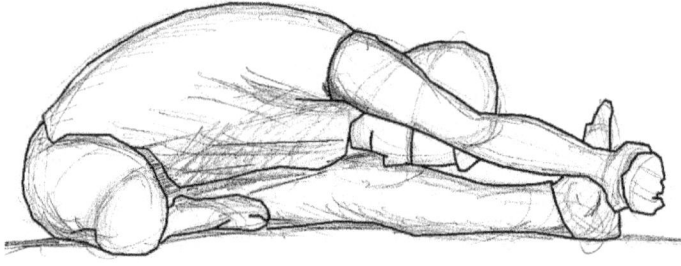

Fig. 9: Head to knee

Spinal Twist:
- Sit with straight legs in front of you.
- Pull the left leg to the center and place the foot under the right leg almost to the buttock.
- Bend the right leg at the knee and place the foot on the floor outside your left thigh. The right knee should point straight up.
- Twist your upper body so that your left shoulder points at the right knee and right shoulder point to the back.
- Place your left hand on the outside thigh of the right leg trying to grab the leg as low as possible.
- The right arm either supports your body. This is the Half Spinal Twist. Stay in it for 5 seconds.
- Repeat on other side.

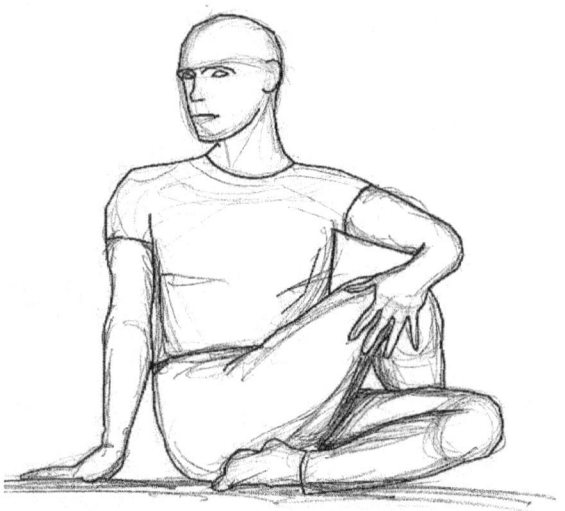

Fig. 10: Spinal Twist

Seated Forward Bend:
- Sit on the floor with your legs straight in front of you.
- Lean forward from the hip joints, not the waist.
- Try to lengthen the front torso into the pose, keeping your head raised.
- Clasp your hands around the ankles and slightly pull into deeper bend.
- Bend the elbows out to the sides.
- Hold for 5 seconds.

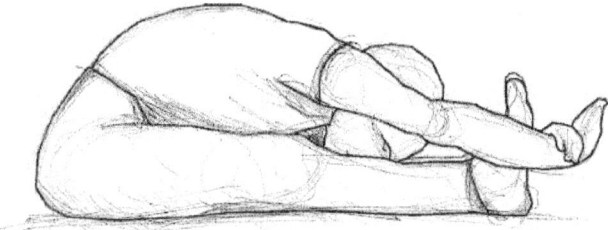

Fig. 11: Forward Bend

Rest or Corpse Pose:
- Lie down. Try to get your body into neutral position.
- Extend your arms alongside your body resting backs of the hands on the floor.
- Let shoulder blades rest evenly on the floor.
- Relax all your muscles.
- Stay in this pose 10-20 seconds.

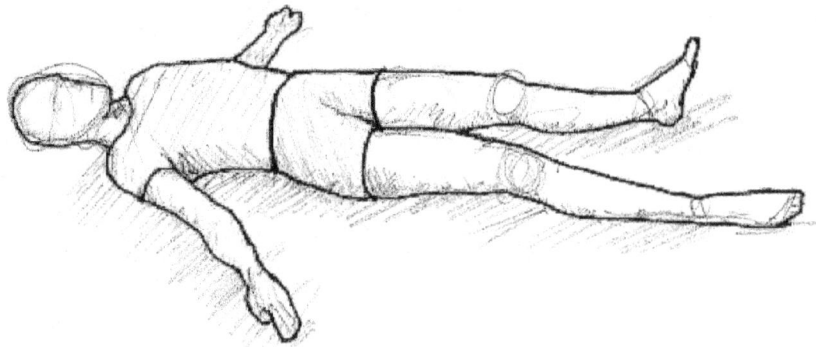

Fig. 12: Corpse Pose

This the end of the routine. It should take you 8 – 10 minutes.

While it may look like not that much, you have an opportunity to observe how your body responds to those poses. Perform those poses slowly. Do not force your bends or twists. Go as far as you can. Remember that you can try to go little farther in the next phase.

Whenever I try to do a new routine I write it down on small piece of paper so I can check if I missed anything. Here is a short **CHECKLIST** (can be found at http://yoga-connect.blogspot.com/) for you:
- Breathing in cross legged sitting position.10 deep breaths.
- Turn your head up & down - 3 times.
- Turn your head left & right - 3 times.
- Clockwise head rotation – twice.
- Counterclockwise head rotation – twice.
- Shoulder shrug your shoulders - 3 times.
- Shoulder stretch - 3 times. Both sides.
- Bow (toe touching) - 2 times.
- Plank Pose (push-up position).
- Cobra Pose - hold 5 seconds.
- Head to the knee with one leg bent - hold 5 seconds. Both sides.
- Spinal Twist - Both sides.
- Seated Forward Bend (head to the knees) hold 5 seconds.
- Corpse Pose (rest) - stay in this pose 10-20 seconds.

Phase 2

This phase will last 3 weeks. Again, please workout 3 days a week.

This time we will introduce an Abdominal Breathing and Sun Salutations. The routine takes 8 minutes (plus/minus).

Abdominal Breathing:
- Sit on the mat in a neutral posture and place your hands on the knees.
- Relax your shoulders.
- Inhale. Feel how your abdomen expand like a balloon. Hold for 2 seconds.
- Slowly contract your abdomen by "sucking" in your belly button - exhale.
- Repeat two-three more times.

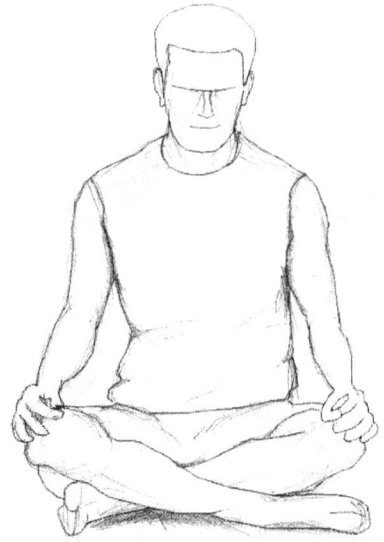

Fig. 13: Neutral Posture

Neck stretching:
- Turn your head up. Look up at the ceiling.
- Turn your head down, "Chin to Chest", look down.
- Repeat, turn your head up.
- Turn your head down.
- Look straight ahead.
- Turn your head 90 degrees to the left.
- Turn back to look straight ahead.

- Turn your head 90 degrees to the right.
- Repeat, turn your head to the left.
- Turn back to look straight ahead.
- Turn your head to the right.
- Look straight ahead. Rest for 2 seconds

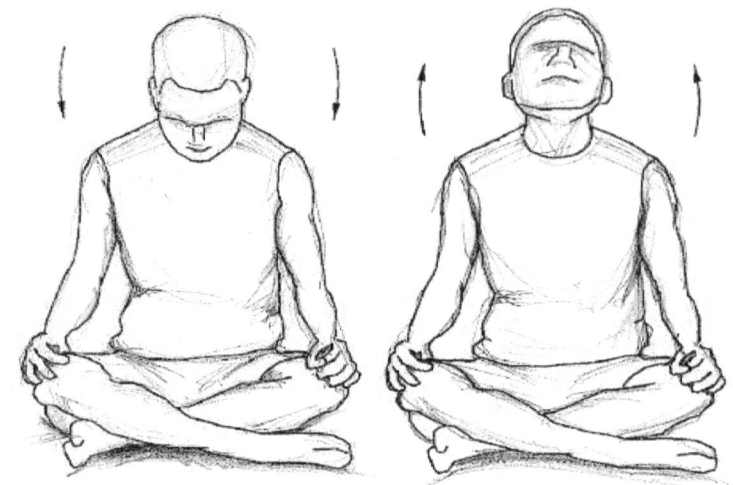

Fig. 14: Head up & down

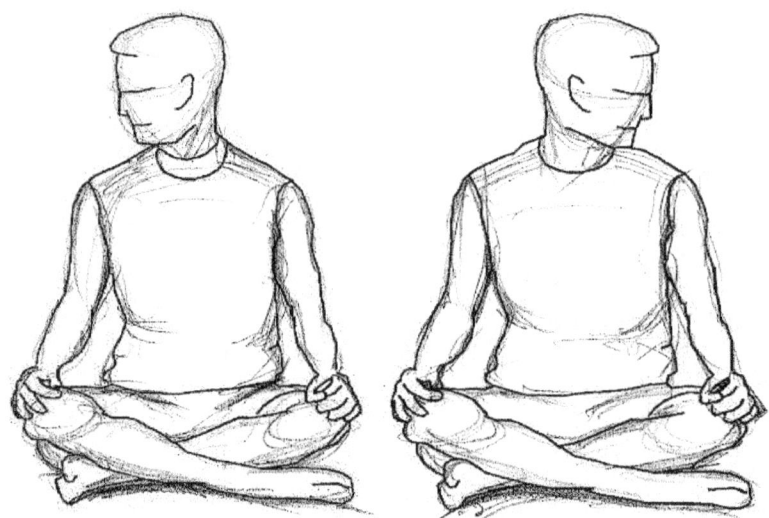

Fig. 15: Head left & right

Neck stretching (continued):
- Gently lower your chin to relax the back of your neck (the only area that is bent is your neck).
- Lower your right ear down towards your shoulder.
- Hold for 2 seconds.
- Return upright.
- Repeat "Ear to Shoulder" on the other side.
- Rest for 2 seconds and repeat the turns two more times.

- Clockwise head rotation – twice.
- Counterclockwise head rotation – twice.

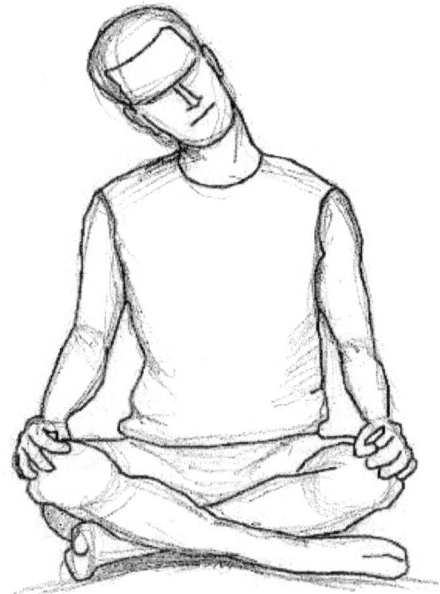

Fig. 16: Ear to Shoulder

Shoulders:
- Shrug your shoulders: while your palms are resting on your knees lift your shoulders and hold for 2 seconds. Let your shoulders drop. Rest for 2 seconds and repeat the shrugs two more times.
- Touch your left ear with your right hand.
- Place your left hand under the elbow of your right hand. Apply pressure on the elbow to force the right hand go far behind your left ear.
- Repeat on the other side.

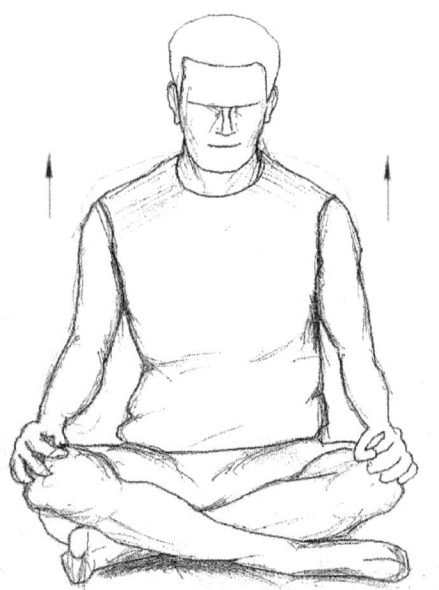

Fig. 17: Shoulder Shrug

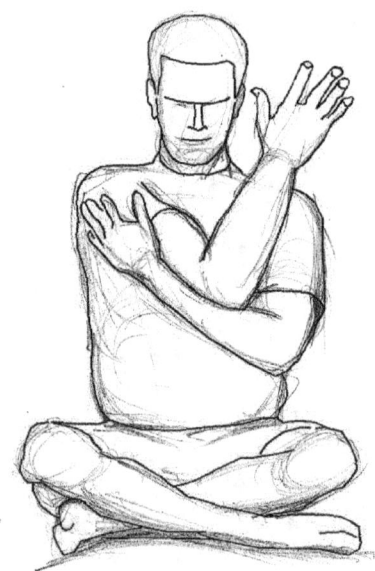

Fig. 18: Shoulder Stretch

Sun Salutation A (two sets):

1. Mountain Pose

   Stand straight with big toes touching (heels can be slightly separated). Distribute weight evenly onto four corners of each foot. Firm you muscles. Gently draw in your belly. Pull back your shoulders.

   - Stand in narrow stance with feet parallel to each other, toes touching.
   - Spread your toes.
   - Distribute your weight evenly on your feet. (You can accomplish that by slowly rocking back and forth.) Let your feet "root down" into the floor.
   - Tighten leg muscles.
   - Pull the shoulders back to open your chest.
   - Take several deep breaths.

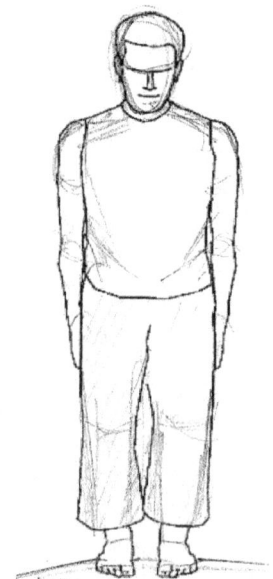

Fig. 19: Mountain Pose

2. Prayer Pose - Exhale

Stand erect with your feet together, exhale. Keep hands joined together, as if you were praying, in front of your chest. Keep your gaze straight ahead.

3. Raised Arms Pose - Inhale
    Inhaling, while keeping your palms together raise your arm arms up over your head until they are straight, look toward hands.

    When you raise your arms don't just raise them, extend them. Extend them farther. You should feel your shoulders being stretched.

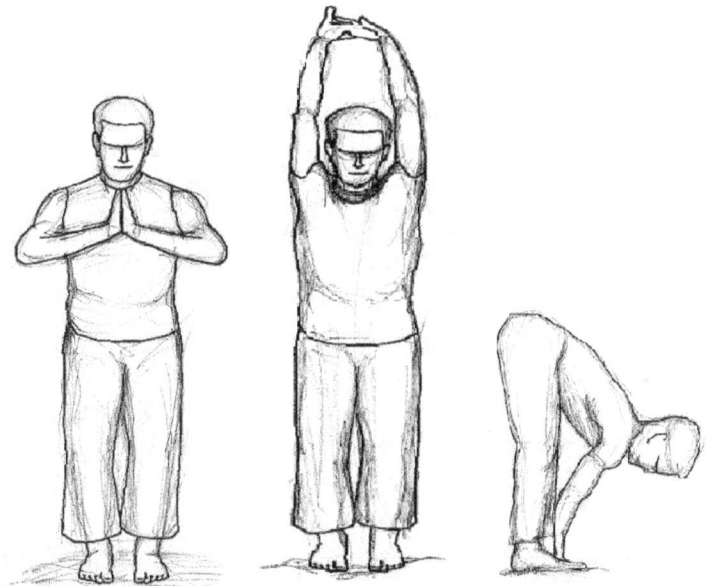

Fig. 20: Prayer - Raised Arms - Half Forward Bend

4. Half Forward Bend Pose - Inhale
    Inhaling, straighten your arms, lift the torso so it is para llel to the floor. Extend and straighten your spine. Place your fingertips on the floor. Look toward a wall in front of you.

    The most important thing in this pose is to keep the spine flat. If you can't place your hands on the floor or you can't do that without curving your back use the blocks under your hands.

5. Plank Pose – hold your breath.
    Place palms on the floor just outside of the feet. Step right foot back into lunge, lower hips. Step your left leg back into push-up position (top of push-up). The arms should be straight and perpendicular to the floor. Shoulders directly over the wrists, torso parallel to the floor. The feet should be on the balls. Backs of your legs and torso should form a straight line.

    This pose strengthens your arms. However, there is a variation of this pose, also called plank, where arms are bent at the elbows (forearms rest on the floor) and it works on abdominal muscles.

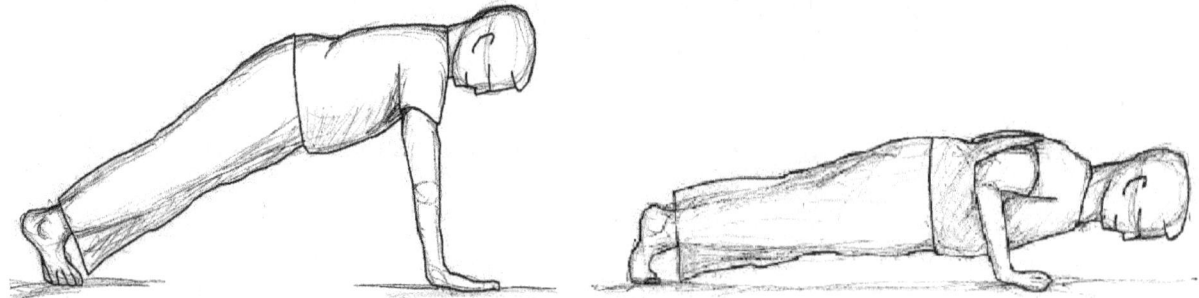

Fig. 21: Plank - Four-Limbed Staff

6. Four-Limbed Staff Pose - Exhale
    Exhaling bend elbows and lower body toward floor until it is 2-3 inches above it (lower push-up position). Gaze down. Hold for 10 seconds.

    Unlike in any other pose, in this pose you will feel that you are using your muscles. You will have to control your descent and then hold your body just off the floor. (If you lower your body slowly to the floor it maybe better then 2-3 pushups.)

7. Cobra Pose - Inhale
    Inhaling, roll your feet over the tips of your toes (the feet may also stay on the balls), lower your hips and thighs toward the floor (touch or almost touch the floor), lift your chest on straight arms. Look straight up.

    This pose will strengthen your spine, stretch the chest, shoulders, and abdomen, firm the buttocks, and relieve stress and fatigue.

8. Downward Dog Pose - Exhale
    Exhaling, push the hips up while rolling your feet back over the tips of your toes. Lift your midsection up. Straighten your legs, try to let your heels touch the floor, stretch out your arms so they are in line with your torso. Look at the floor. Hold.

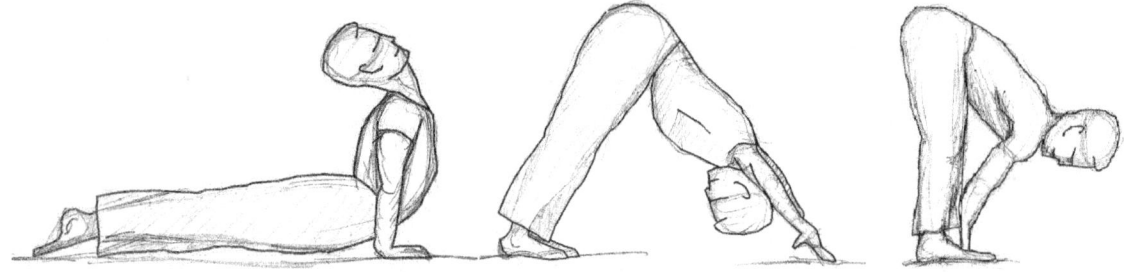

Fig. 22: Cobra - Downward Dog - Half Forward Bend

9. Half Forward Bend Pose - Inhale
    Look up between your hands. Inhaling step right foot up between your hands, then step your left foot in next to your right foot. Straighten your arms and legs. The torso should be parallel to the floor. Place your fingertips on the floor. Look straight forward.

10. Forward Bend Pose - Exhale

While exhaling: lower your torso toward floor keeping the spine straight. Place your fingertips on the floor just outside your feet. The fingertips should be aligned with your toes. Bring the torso and head toward your legs in forward fold.

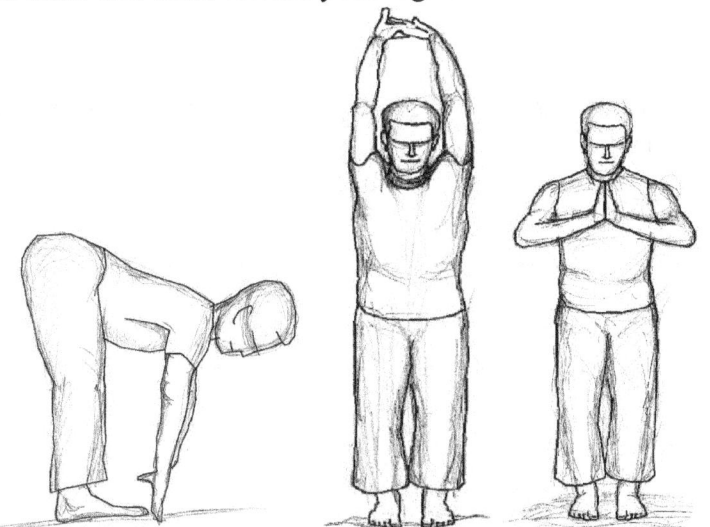

Fig. 23: Forward Bend - Raised Arms - Prayer

11. Raised Arms Pose - Inhale
    While inhaling: lift your torso up to the standing position, sweep your arms up overhead, the palms come together.

12. Return to Prayer Pose - Exhale
    Lower the hands in front of your chest to the prayer position.
    Then, release the arms by the sides of your body.

13. REPEAT.

Head to the Knee:

- Sit with straight legs in front of you.
- Pull the left leg to the center and place the foot sole lightly against the inner thigh of the right leg so the shin is at a right angle to the right leg.
- While holding the left ankle with the left hand grab the right ankle with the other hand. Pull your head to the right knee.
- This is the Head to Knee Pose. Stay in it for 5 seconds.
- Repeat on other side.

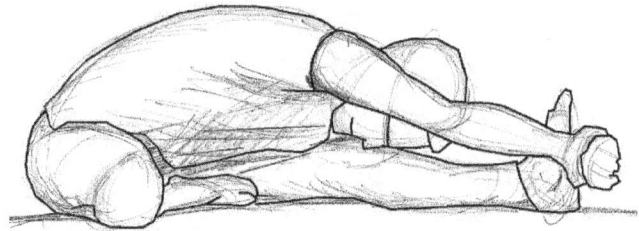

Fig. 24: Head to knee

Spinal Twist:
- Sit with straight legs in front of you.
- Pull the left leg to the center and place the foot under the right leg almost to the buttock.
- Bend the right leg at the knee and place the foot on the floor outside your left thigh. The right knee should point straight up.
- Twist your upper body so that your left shoulder points at the right knee and right shoulder point to the back.
- Place your left hand on the outside thigh of the right leg trying to grab the leg as low as possible.
- The right arm either supports your body. This is the Half Spinal Twist. Stay in it for 5 seconds.
- Repeat on other side.

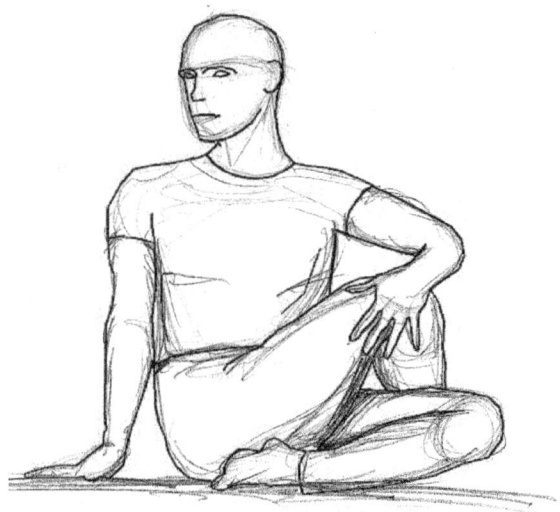

Fig. 25: Spinal Twist

Seated Forward Bend:
- Sit on the floor with your legs straight in front of you.
- Lean forward from the hip joints, not the waist.
- Try to lengthen the front torso into the pose, keeping your head raised.
- Clasp your hands around the ankles and slightly pull into deeper bend.
- Bend the elbows out to the sides.
- Hold for 5 seconds.

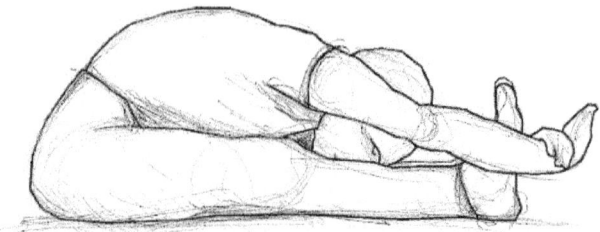

Fig. 26: Forward Bend

Rest or Corpse Pose:
- Lie down. Try to get your body into neutral position.
- Extend your arms alongside your body resting backs of the hands on the floor.
- Let shoulder blades rest evenly on the floor.
- Relax all your muscles.
- Stay in this pose 10-20 seconds.

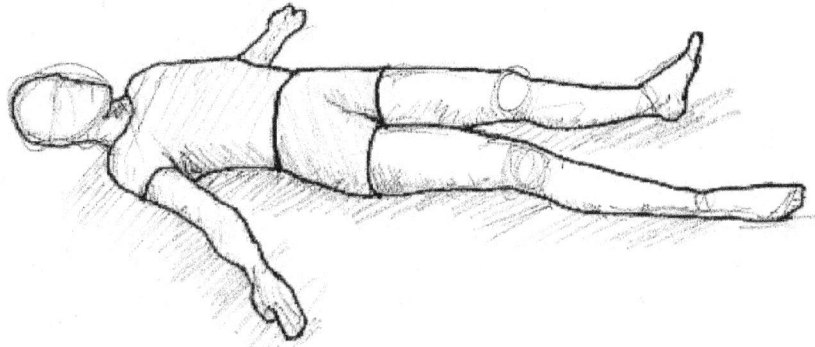

Fig. 27: Corpse Pose

This the end of the routine. It should take you 8 minutes.

Phase 2 checklist can be found at: http://yoga-connect.blogspot.com/

Phase 3

This phase will last 2 months. Unless you have another activity every other day, you can start working out 6 days a week. Take a break on the seventh day. We are adding more exercises including second Sun Salutation. This routine takes +/- 15 minutes.

Abdominal Breathing:
- Sit on the mat in a neutral posture and place your hands on the knees.
- Relax your shoulders.
- Inhale. Feel how your abdomen expand like a balloon. Hold for 2 seconds.
- Slowly contract your abdomen by "sucking" in your belly button - exhale.
- Repeat two-three more times.

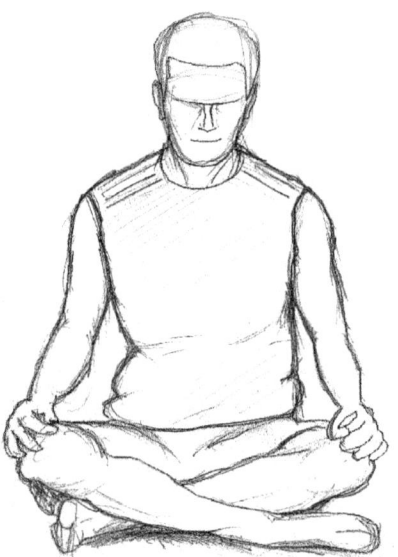

Fig. 28: Neutral Posture

Neck stretching:
- Turn your head up. Look up at the ceiling.
- Turn your head down, "Chin to Chest", look down.
- Repeat, turn your head up.
- Turn your head down.
- Look straight ahead.
- Turn your head 90 degrees to the left.
- Turn back to look straight ahead.
- Turn your head 90 degrees to the right.

- Repeat, turn your head to the left.
- Turn back to look straight ahead.
- Turn your head to the right.
- Look straight ahead. Rest for 2 seconds

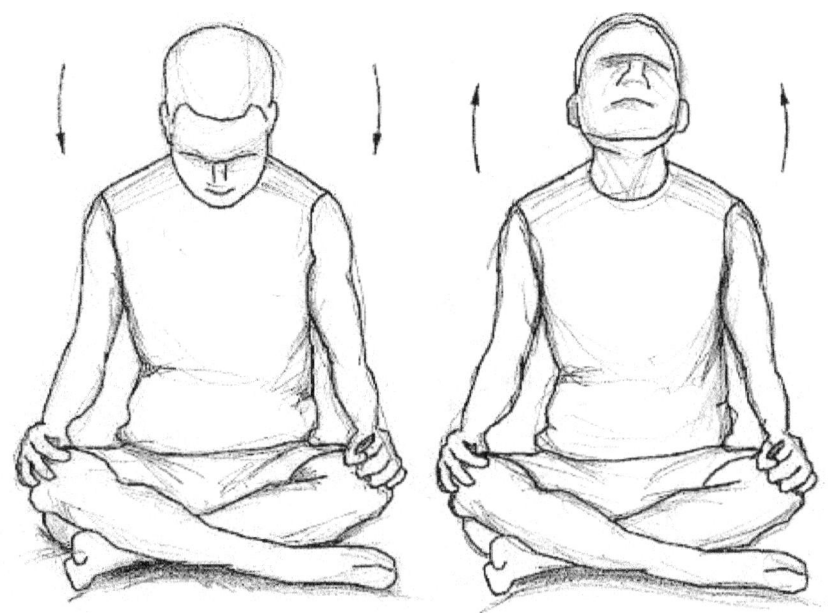

Fig. 29: Head up & down

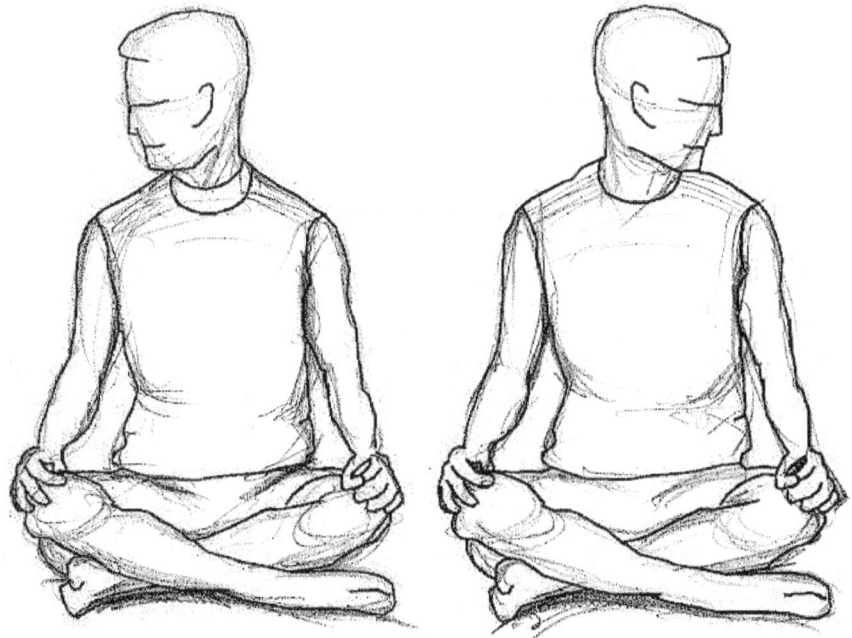

Fig. 30: Head left & right

Neck stretching (continued):
- Gently lower your chin to relax the back of your neck (the only area that is bent is your neck).
- Lower your right ear down towards your shoulder.
- Hold for 2 seconds.
- Return upright.
- Repeat "Ear to Shoulder" on the other side.
- Rest for 2 seconds and repeat the turns two more times.
- Clockwise head rotation – twice.
- Counterclockwise head rotation – twice.

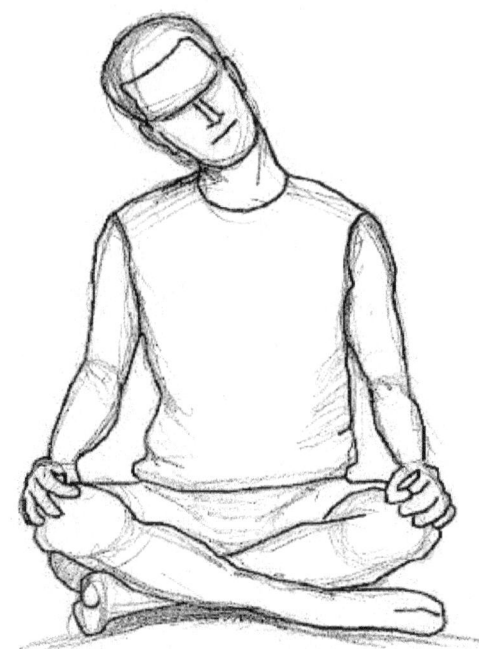

Fig. 31: Ear to Shoulder

Shoulders:
- Shrug your shoulders: while your palms are resting on your knees lift your shoulders and hold for 2 seconds. Let your shoulders drop. Rest for 2 seconds and repeat the shrugs two more times.
- Touch your left ear with your right hand.
- Place your left hand under the elbow of your right hand. Apply pressure on the elbow to force the right hand go far behind your left ear.
- Repeat on the other side.

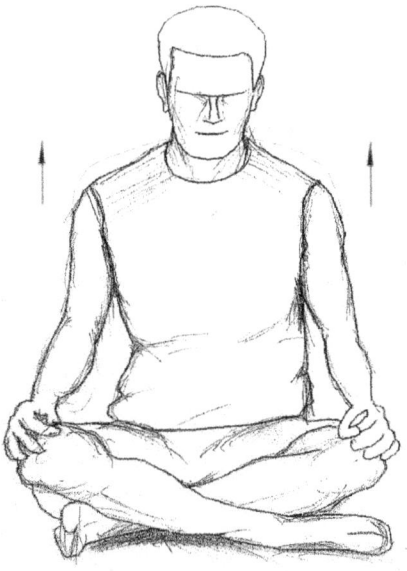

Fig. 32: Shoulder Shrug

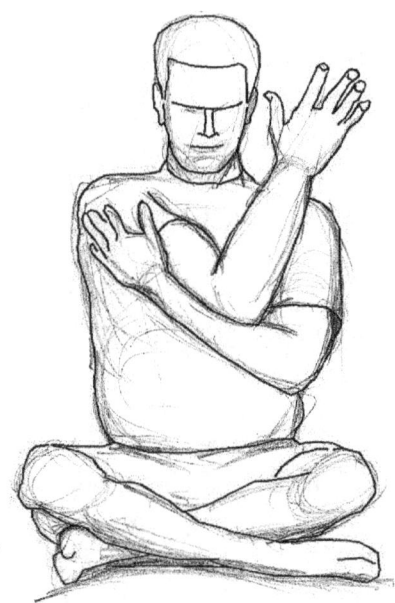

Fig. 33: Shoulder Stretch

Half Back-roll (roll like a ball)
-- If you have any back problems, recent injuries or surgeries, talk to your doctor about this exercise! --
Both Yoga and Pilates have an exercise that we can call "roll like a ball" however, the exercise I propose is based on Aikido warm-up exercise used to teach students how to do back-rollover. The exercise is nearly identical (but better) to the ones practiced in Yoga and Pilates but for one detail that makes it easier and safer to perform. (Aikido practitioners have this one perfected because 80% of their practice is rollovers and brake-falls.) I call it half back-roll because you stop half way (yes, you could go all the way so, be careful) and come back. This exercise is a great back massage.

In Yoga/Pilates, when you roll your body is straight and you roll on your spine. In Aikido your body is off-centered, enough to prevent you from rolling on the spine. While in Yoga and Pilates you will feel this roll, in Aikido the discomfort is minimal.

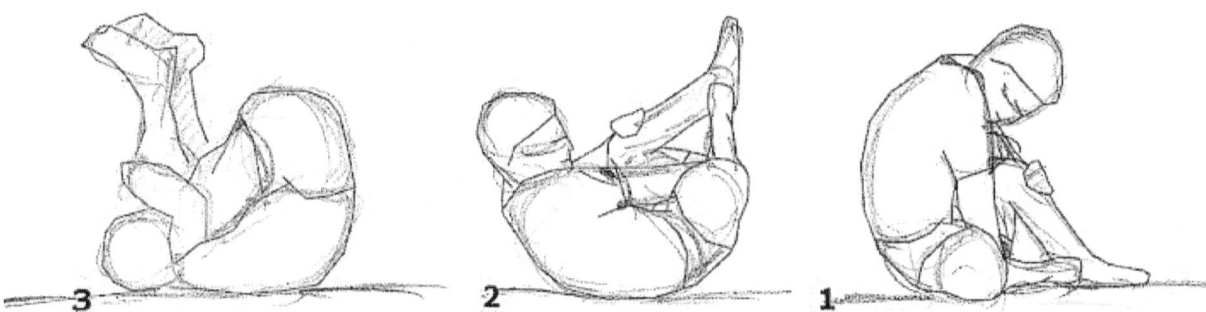

Fig. 34: Back-roll

- Sit on the mat (required – first few times you may use 2 mats) with both legs bent at the knees. One leg is turned so the sides of the thigh and the knee rest on the floor. The knee of the other leg is pointed up and foot is flat on the floor. Keep your chin pressed to your chest.
- Push-off with your front leg and slowly roll on your back.
- When your legs are above your head (and area touching the floor is between your shoulder blades - #3) stop the motion.
- Come back to the original position but switch legs on the way back.
- Stop. Get ready to push-off with the other leg.
- Repeat three (3) more times changing legs on the way back.

Notes:
1. Stop the backward roll when you reach the area between your shoulder blades. While your head and neck will touch the mat they should not get compressed against it.
2. Make your rolling motion smooth.
3. Keep your chin pressed to your chest through out the whole motion.

Sun Salutation A (two sets):
1. Mountain Pose
   Stand straight with big toes touching (heels can be slightly separated). Distribute weight evenly onto four corners of each foot. Firm you muscles. Gently draw in your belly. Pull back your shoulders.
   - Stand in narrow stance with feet parallel to each other, toes touching.
   - Spread your toes.
   - Distribute your weight evenly on your feet. (You can accomplish that by slowly rocking back and forth.) Let your feet "root down" into the floor.
   - Tighten leg muscles.
   - Pull the shoulders back to open your chest.

- Take several deep breaths.

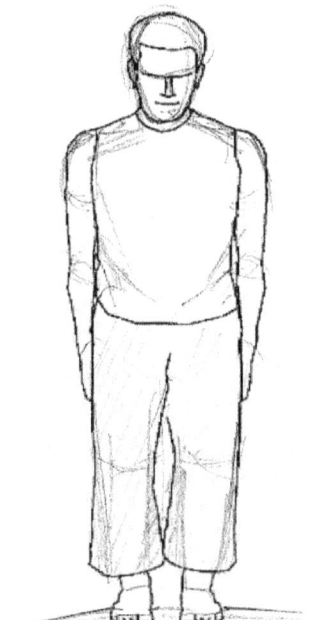

Fig. 35: Mountain Pose

2. Prayer Pose - Exhale
   Stand erect with your feet together, exhale. Keep hands joined together, as if you were praying, in front of your chest. Keep your gaze straight ahead.

3. Raised Arms Pose - Inhale
   Inhaling, while keeping your palms together raise your arm arms up over your head until they are straight, look toward hands.

   When you raise your arms don't just raise them, extend them. Extend them farther. You should feel your shoulders being stretched.

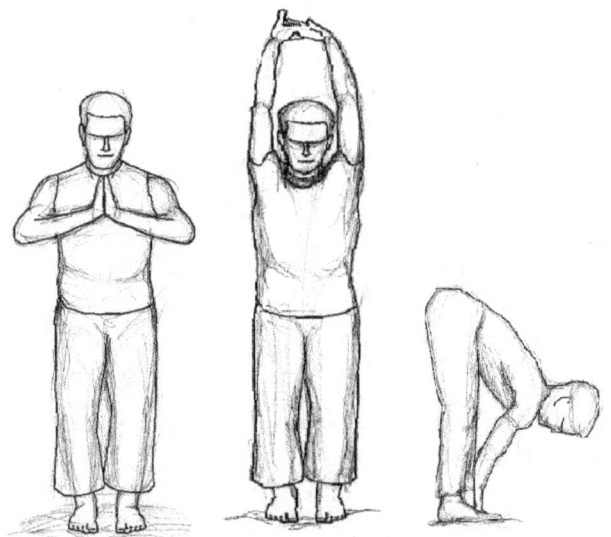

Fig. 36: Prayer - Raised Arms - Half Forward Bend poses

4. Half Forward Bend Pose - Inhale
    Inhaling, straighten your arms, lift the torso so it is para llel to the floor. Extend and straighten your spine. Place your fingertips on the floor. Look toward a wall in front of you.

    The most important thing in this pose is to keep the spine flat. If you can't place your hands on the floor or you can't do that without curving your back use the blocks under your hands.

5. Plank Pose – hold your breath.
    Place palms on the floor just outside of the feet. Step right foot back into lunge, lower hips. Step your left leg back into push-up position (top of push-up). The arms should be straight and perpendicular to the floor. Shoulders directly over the wrists, torso parallel to the floor. The feet should be on the balls. Backs of your legs and torso should form a straight line.

    This pose strengthens your arms. However, there is a variation of this pose, also called plank, where arms are bent at the elbows (forearms rest on the floor) and it works on abdominal muscles.

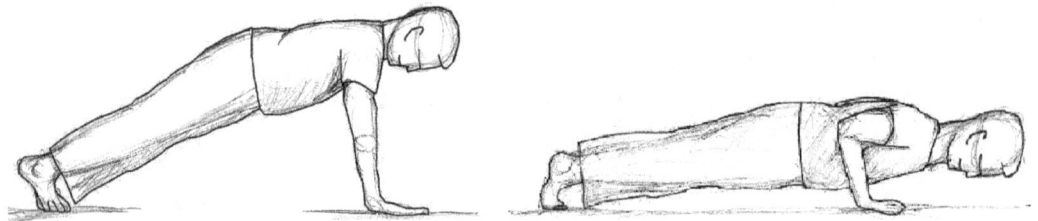

Fig. 37: Plank - Four-Limbed Staff poses

6. Four-Limbed Staff Pose - Exhale
    Exhaling bend elbows and lower body toward floor until it is 2-3 inches above it (lower push-up position). Gaze down. Hold for 10 seconds.

    Unlike in any other pose, in this pose you will feel that you are using your muscles. You will have to control your descent and then hold your body just off the floor. (If you lower your body slowly to the floor it maybe better then 2-3 pushups.)

7. Cobra Pose - Inhale
    Inhaling, roll your feet over the tips of your toes (the feet may also stay on the balls), lower your hips and thighs toward the floor (touch or almost touch the floor), lift your chest on straight arms. Look straight up.

    This pose will strengthen your spine, stretch the chest, shoulders, and abdomen, firm the buttocks, and relieve stress and fatigue.

8. Downward Dog Pose (Adho Mukha Svanasana) - Exhale
    Exhaling, push the hips up while rolling your feet back over the tips of your toes. Lift

your midsection up. Straighten your legs, try to let your heels touch the floor, stretch out your arms so they are in line with your torso. Look at the floor. Hold.

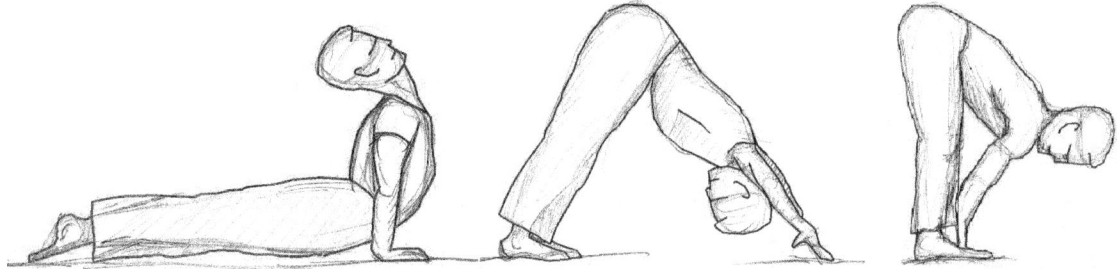

Fig. 38: Cobra - Downward Dog - Half Forward Bend poses

9. Half Forward Bend Pose - Inhale
   Look up between your hands. Inhaling step right foot up between your hands, then step your left foot in next to your right foot. Straighten your arms and legs. The torso should be parallel to the floor. Place your fingertips on the floor. Look straight forward.

10. Forward Bend Pose - Exhale
    While exhaling: lower your torso toward floor keeping the spine straight. Place your fingertips on the floor just outside your feet. The fingertips should be aligned with your toes. Bring the torso and head toward your legs in forward fold.

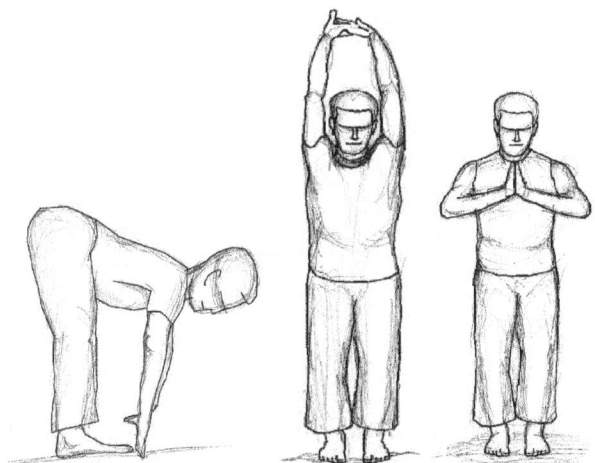

Fig. 39: Forward Bend - Raised Arms – Prayer poses

11. Raised Arms Pose - Inhale
    While inhaling: lift your torso up to the standing position, sweep your arms up overhead, the palms come together.

12. Return to Prayer Pose - Exhale
    Lower the hands in front of your chest to the prayer position.
    Then, release the arms by the sides of your body.

Sun Salutation B (two sets)
Sun Salutation B is a longer sequence of movements then Sun Salutation A. It builds up heat within the body. If you are doing it with intensity, you will break sweat.

1. Prayer Pose - Exhale
   Standing erect with feet together, exhale. Keep hands joined together, as if you were praying, in front of your chest. Keep your gaze straight ahead.

2. Raise your hands over the head – hold your breath.

3. Chair Pose - Inhale
   Inhaling, bend knees, lower hips until thighs are almost parallel to the floor. Sweep arms out and up toward the ceiling, palms face in, bring torso more vertical into Chair pose. This is a deep squat pose. It engages your legs, back, and ankles. If you are a skier you will see its benefits better then anyone.

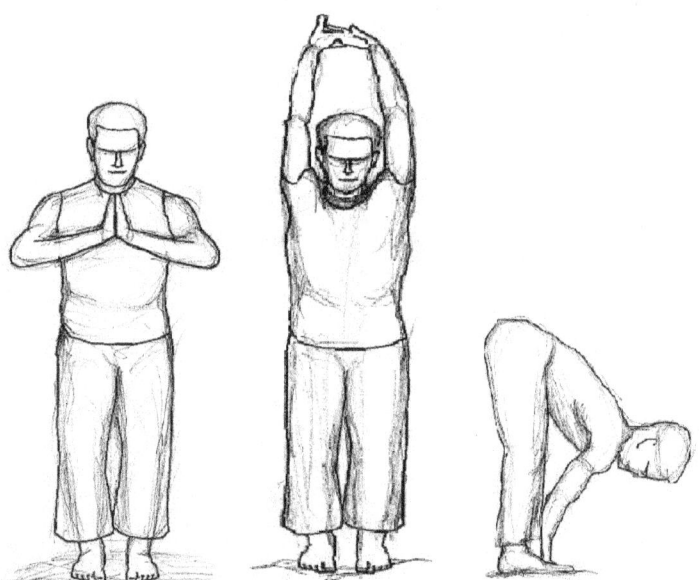

Fig. 40: Prayer - Chair poses

4. Forward Bend Pose – Exhale
   While exhaling: keeping the spine straight lower your torso toward the floor, place your fingertips on the floor just outside your feet, the fingertips should be in line with the toes. Bring the torso and head toward legs in a forward fold. Try to place your hands flat on the floor.

5. Half Forward Bend Pose - Inhale
   Inhaling, straighten your arms, lift the torso so it is parallel to the floor. Extend and straighten your spine. Place your fingertips on the floor. Look toward a wall in front of you. Place palms on the floor just outside of feet (transition). Step right foot back into lunge, lower hips. Step your left leg back into pushup position (top of pushup position). The arms should be perpendicular to the floor. The feet should be on the balls. Backs of your legs and torso should form a straight line.

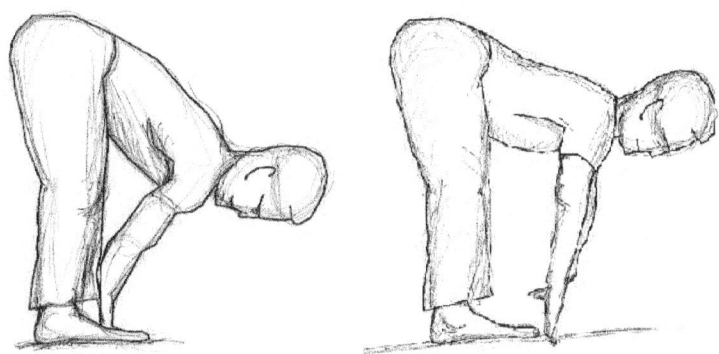

Fig. 41: Forward Bend - Half Forward Bend poses

6. Plank Pose - Transition
    Place palms on the floor just outside of the feet. Step right foot back into lunge, lower
    hips. Step your left leg back into push-up position (top of push-up). The arms should be
    perpendicular to the floor. The feet should be on the balls. Backs of your legs and torso
    should form a straight line.

    This pose strengthens your arms. However, there is a variation of this pose, also called
    plank, were arms are bent at the elbows (forearms rest on the floor) and it works on
    abdominal muscles.

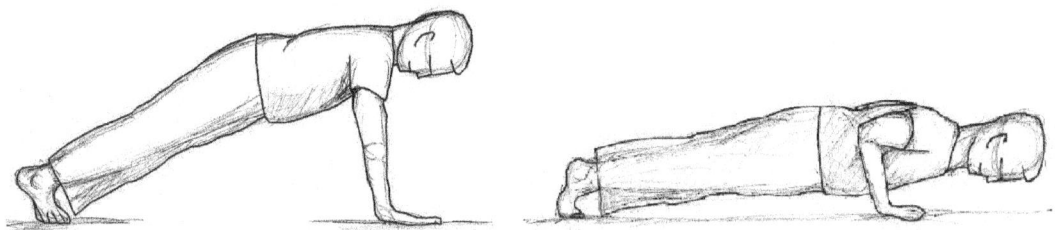

Fig. 42: Plank - Four-Limbed Staff poses

7. Four-Limbed Staff Pose - Exhale
    Exhaling bend elbows and lower body toward floor until you almost touch it (lower push-
    up position). Gaze down. Hold for 10 seconds.

8. Cobra Pose - Inhale
    Inhaling, roll your feet over the tips of your toes (the feet may also stay on the balls),
    lower your hips and thighs toward the floor (touch or almost touch the floor), lift your
    chest on straight arms. Look straight up.

9. Downward Dog Pose - Exhale
    Exhaling, push the hips up while rolling your feet back over the tips of your toes. Lift
    your midsection up. Straighten your legs, try to let your heels touch the floor, stretch out
    your arms so they are in line with your torso. Look at the floor. Hold.

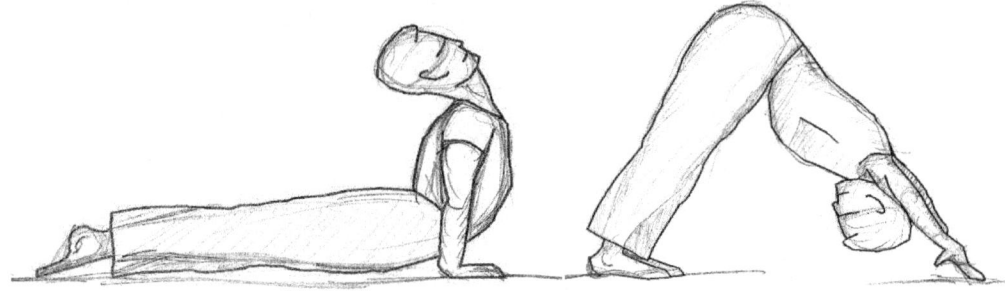

Fig. 43: Cobra - Downward Dog poses

10. Warrior I Pose - Inhale
    While inhaling make a step with your right leg. Raise your hands above the head. Bring palms together. Gaze at the thumbs. Hold for 10 seconds. Slightly bend your knees, step back into Plank.
    The pose strengthens the legs (long step) and opens the chest.

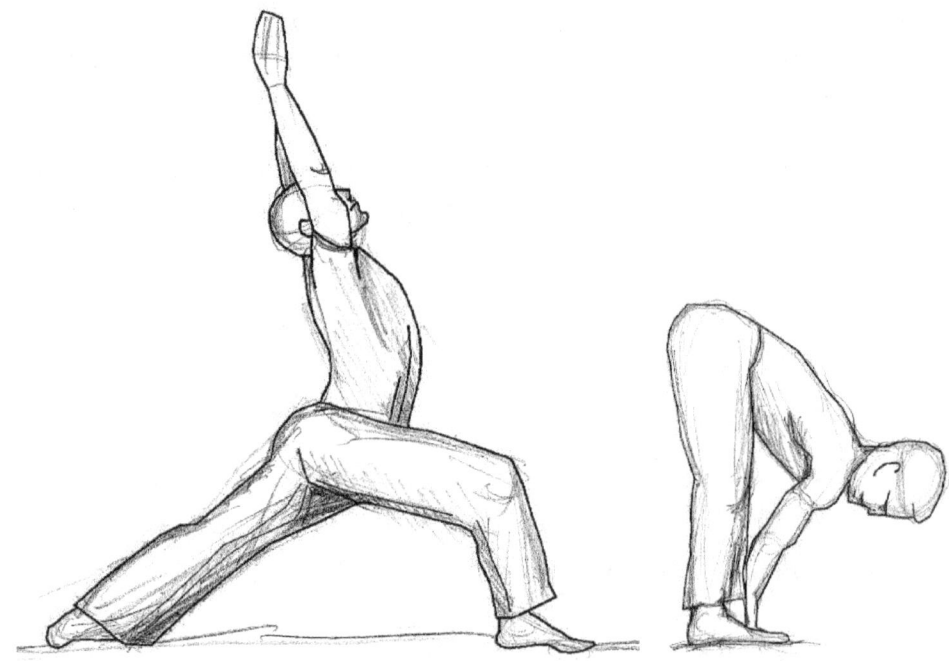

Fig. 44: Warrior I - Forward Bend poses

11. Forward Bend Pose – Exhale
    While exhaling: keeping the spine straight lower your torso toward the floor, place your fingertips on the floor just outside your feet, the fingertips should be in line with the toes. Bring the torso and head toward legs in a forward fold. Try to place your hands flat on the floor.
    This pose can be used as a resting position between the standing poses. Stay in the pose for 10 seconds.

12. Half Forward Bend Pose - Inhale
    Inhaling, straighten your arms, lift the torso so it is parallel to the floor. Extend and straighten your spine. Place your fingertips on the floor. Look toward a wall in front of you. Place palms on the floor just outside of feet (transition). Step right foot back into

lunge, lower hips. Step your left leg back into pushup position (top of pushup position). The arms should be perpendicular to the floor. The feet should be on the balls. Backs of your legs and torso should form a straight line

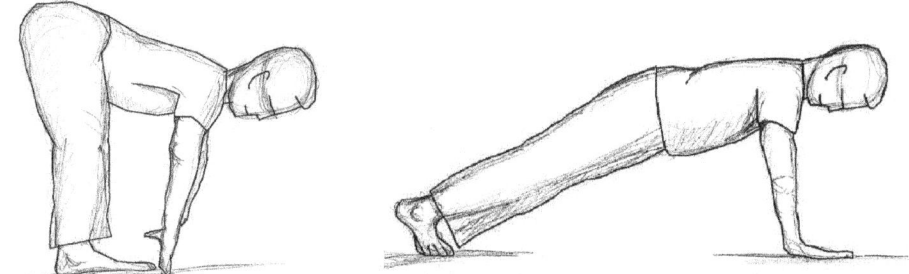

Fig. 45: Half Forward Bend - Plank poses

13. Plank Pose - Transition
    Place palms on the floor just outside of the feet. Step right foot back into lunge, lower hips. Step your left leg back into push-up position (top of push-up). The arms should be perpendicular to the floor. The feet should be on the balls. Backs of your legs and torso should form a straight line.

14. Four-Limbed Staff Pose - Exhale
    Exhaling bend elbows and lower body toward floor almost touching it. Gaze down. Hold for 10 seconds.

15. Cobra Pose - Inhale
    Inhaling, roll your feet over the tips of your toes (the feet may also stay on the balls), lower your hips and thighs toward the floor (touch or almost touch the floor), lift your chest on straight arms. Look straight up.

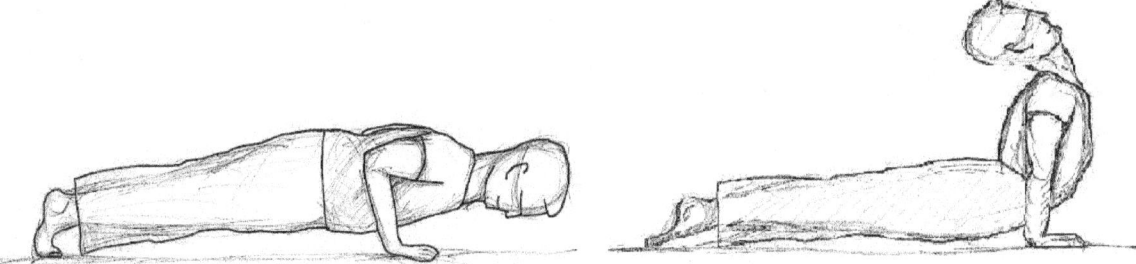

Fig. 46: Four-Limbed Staff – Cobra poses

16. Downward Dog Pose - Exhale
    Exhaling, push the hips up while rolling your feet back over the tips of your toes. Lift your midsection up. Straighten your legs, try to let your heels touch the floor, stretch out your arms so they are in line with your torso. Look at the floor. Hold.

17. Begin inhaling as you look up between hands. Step left foot up between hands.

18. Warrior I Pose - Inhale
    Continue inhaling as you rise into Warrior Pose. Sweep arms overhead. Bring palms together. Gaze at the thumbs.

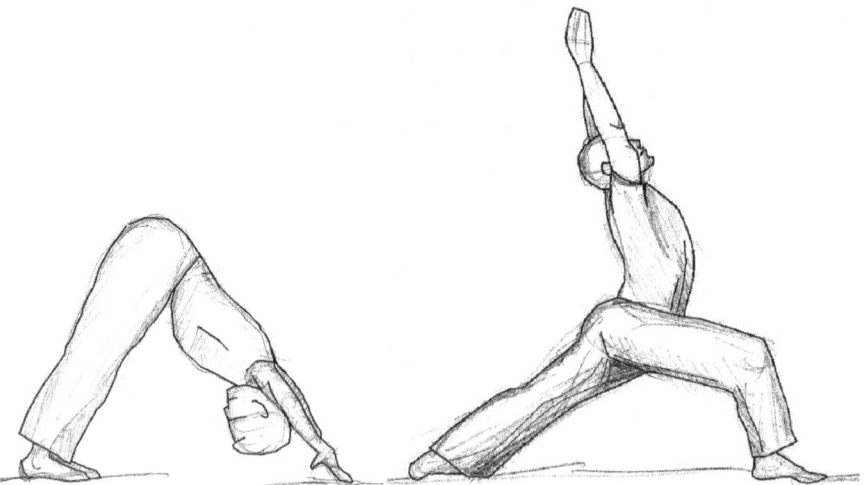

Fig. 47: Downward - Warrior I poses

19. Forward Bend Pose – Exhale

    While exhaling: keeping the spine straight lower your torso toward the floor, place your fingertips on the floor just outside your feet, the fingertips should be in line with the toes. Bring the torso and head toward legs in a forward fold. Try to place your hands flat on the floor.

    This pose can be used as a resting position between the standing poses. Stay in the pose for 30 seconds to 1 minute.

20. Half Forward Bend Pose - Inhale

    Inhaling, straighten your arms, lift the torso so it is parallel to the floor. Extend and straighten your spine. Place your fingertips on the floor. Look toward a wall in front of you. Place palms on the floor just outside of feet (transition). Step right foot back into lunge, lower hips. Step your left leg back into pushup position (top of pushup position). The arms should be perpendicular to the floor. The feet should be on the balls. Backs of your legs and torso should form a straight line.

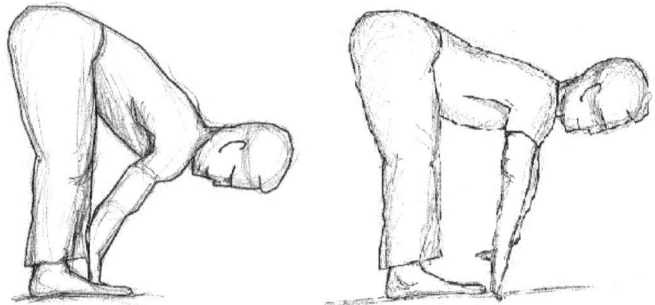

Fig. 48: Forward & Half Forward Bend poses

21. Plank Pose - Transition

    Place palms on the floor just outside of the feet. Step right foot back into lunge, lower hips. Step your left leg back into push-up position (top of push-up). The arms should be perpendicular to the floor. The feet should be on the balls. Backs of your legs and torso should form a straight line.

22. Four-Limbed Staff Pose - Exhale
    Exhaling place palms on the floor. Step back into the Plank Pose. Exhaling bend elbows and lower body toward floor. Gaze down. Hold for 10 seconds.

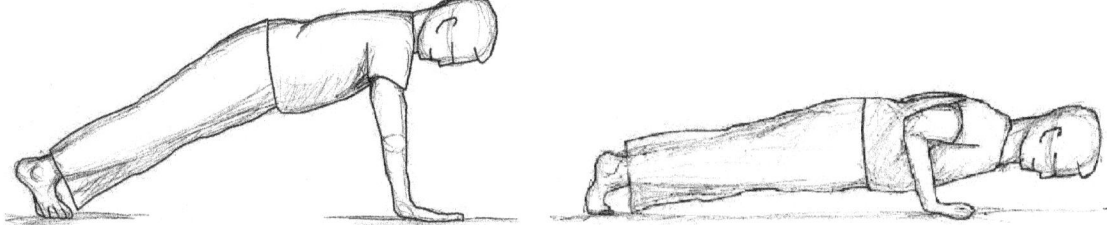

Fig. 49: Plank & Four Limbed Staff poses

23. Cobra Pose - Inhale
    Inhaling, roll your feet over the tips of your toes (the feet may also stay on the balls), lower your hips and thighs toward the floor touch or almost touch the floor), lift your chest on straight arms. Look straight up. (Fig. 46).

24. Downward Dog Pose - Exhale
    Exhaling, push the hips up while rolling your feet back over the tips of your toes. Lift your midsection up. Straighten your legs, try to let your heels touch the floor, stretch out your arms so they are in line with your torso. Look at the floor. Hold.

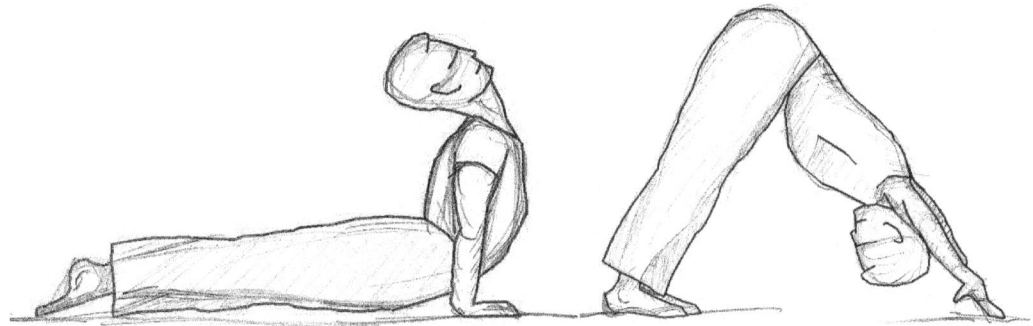

Fig. 50: Cobra & Downward Dog Poses

25. Begin inhaling as you look up between hands. Step left foot up between hands.

26. Half Forward Bend Pose - Inhale
    Look up between your hands. Inhaling step right foot up between your hands, then step your left foot in next to your right foot. Straighten your legs and arms. The torso should be parallel to the floor. Place your fingertips on the floor. Look straight forward.

27. Forward Bend Pose - Exhale
    Inhaling, straighten your arms, lift the torso so it is parallel to the floor. Extend and straighten your spine. Place your fingertips on the floor. Look toward a wall in front of you. Bring the torso and head toward your legs in forward fold.

28. Chair Pose - Inhale
   Inhaling, bend knees, lower hips until thighs are almost parallel to the floor. Sweep arms

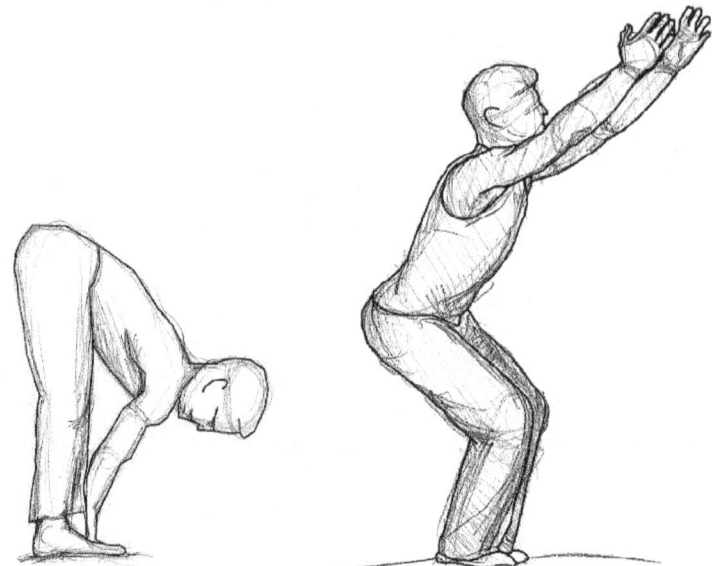

Fig. 51: Forward Bend & Chair Poses

out and up toward the ceiling, palms face in, bring torso more vertical into Chair pose.

29. Raised Arms Pose - Hold breath
   While inhaling: lift your torso up to the standing position, sweep your arms up overhead, the palms come together.

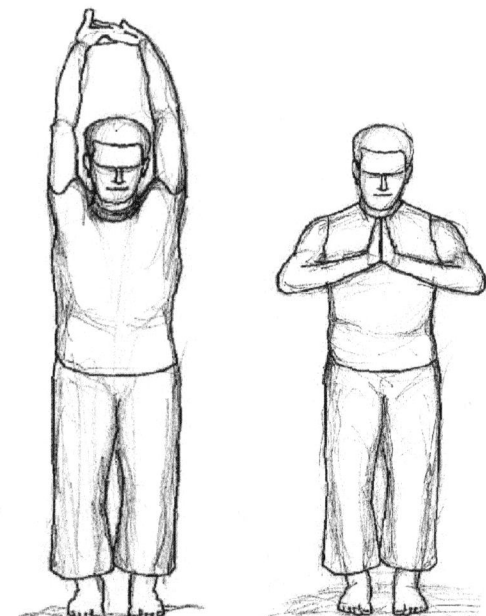

Fig. 52: Raised Arms & Prayer Poses

30. Prayer Pose - Exhale
   Exhale and straighten your legs. Lower the arms to your chest, Prayer Pose.

Tree Pose
- Start with a Mountain Pose.
- Shift your weight onto your left foot, bend your right knee and lift your right foot bringing it to the center.
- Place the sole of your right foot on the inner left thigh. You can start right above the knee. As you are more comfortable, you can progress to the point where you cannot bring your leg any higher.
- Press your palms together in front of your chest and raise them above your head. Look straight ahead.

(If you need to support your pose you can hold your leg with one hand, preferably from the same side, and raise the other hand over your head.)
Stay in the Tree Pose from 10 seconds to 20 seconds. Repeat on the other side.

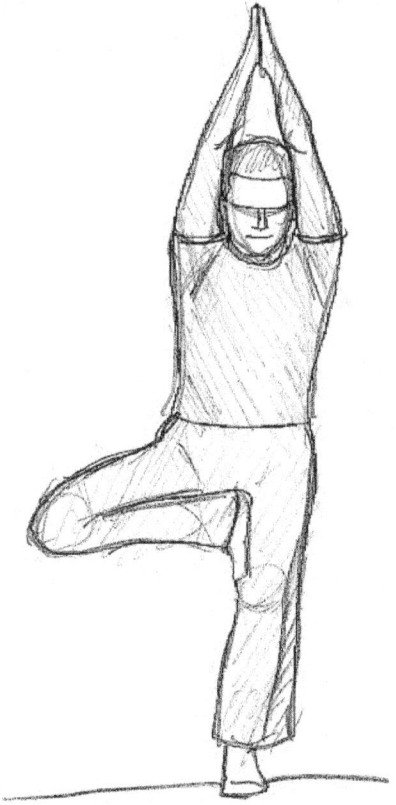

Fig. 53: Tree Pose

Superman Pose
1. Lie face-down on the floor, feet together, chin on the floor.
2. Stretch the arms in front of you as far as you can.
3. Breathing in, raise the upper torso, arms, and legs. Keep your elbows and knees straight.
4. Hold and continue with long, gentle breaths (in and out). Breathing out, release and relax.

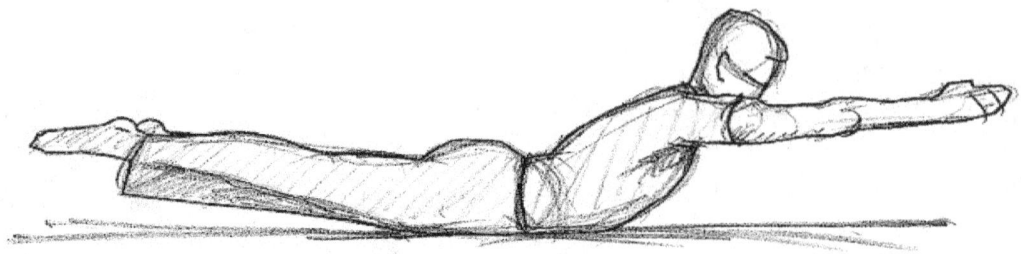

Fig. 54: Superman Pose

Benefits:
Tones the arms and legs. Strengthens abdominal muscles and lower back.

Locust Pose
- Lie on your belly with your arms along the sides of your torso, palms up.
- Rotate your thighs by turning your big toes toward each other. Firm your buttocks.
- Exhale and lift your head, upper torso, arms, and legs away from the floor.
- Raise your arms parallel to the floor and stretch them back through your fingertips.
- Gaze forward or slightly upward.

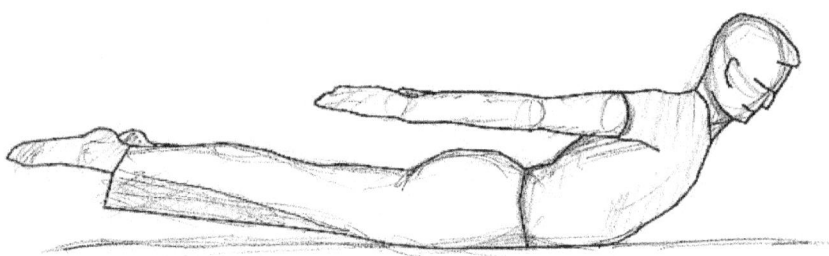

Fig. 55: Locust Pose

Stay in the pose from 10 seconds to 20 seconds, then release with an exhalation. Take a breath and repeat 1 or 2 times.

Bridge Pose
- Lie down on the floor. Arms on the sides.
- Bend your knees and place your feet firmly on the floor as close to your buttocks as possible.
- Lift your hips off the floor. Keep your arms flat on the floor. Your feet and thighs should be parallel, 4 - 6 inches apart. Lift your hips as much as you can. The knees should be directly over the heels. Your spine should arch so you much that only top your shoulder, neck and back of your head touch the floor.

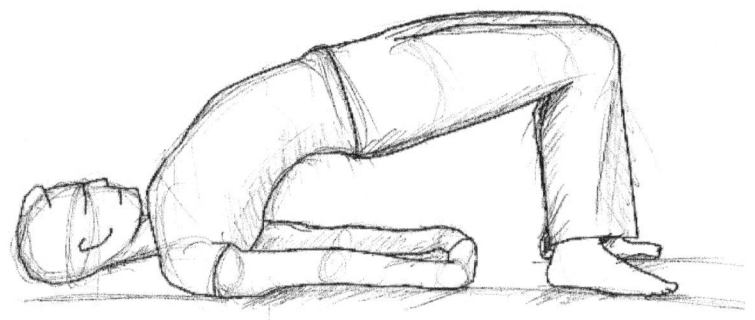

Fig. 56: Bridge Pose

Stay in the Bridge Pose for 10 seconds or little more. When you release from the pose roll the spine down slowly onto the floor.

Half Boat Pose
- Lie supine on the mat.
- Lift your legs 6 inches above the floor.
- Lift your upper body 6 inches above the floor with hands along the body. Hold for 30 seconds. Both legs and upper body are only a half the distance from the floor, hence… Half Boat Pose. Hold it for 10 seconds.

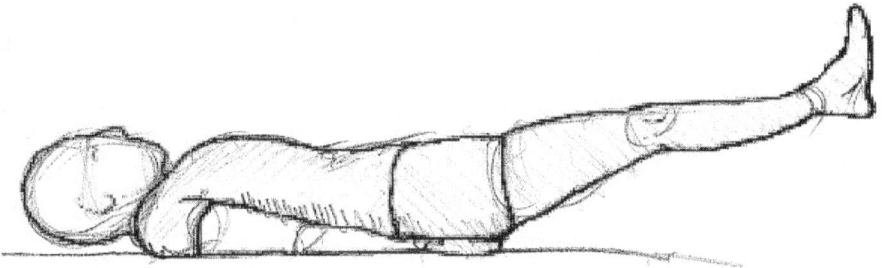

Fig. 57: Half Boat Pose

Head to the Knee:
- Sit with straight legs in front of you.
- Pull the left leg to the center and place the foot sole lightly against the inner thigh of the right leg so the shin is at a right angle to the right leg.
- While holding the left ankle with the left hand grab the right ankle with the other hand. Pull your head to the right knee. Hold for 5-10 seconds.
- Repeat on other side.

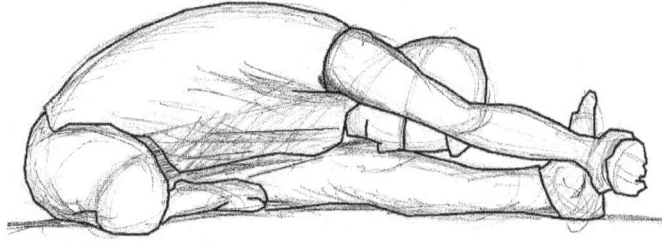

Fig. 58: Head to knee

Spinal Twist:
- Sit with straight legs in front of you.
- Pull the left leg to the center and place the foot under the right leg almost to the buttock.
- Bend the right leg at the knee and place the foot on the floor outside your left thigh. The right knee should point straight up.
- Twist your upper body so that your left shoulder points at the right knee and right shoulder point to the back.
- Place your left hand on the outside thigh of the right leg trying to grab the leg as low as possible.
- The right arm either supports your body. This is the Half Spinal Twist. Stay in it for 5 seconds.
- Repeat on other side.

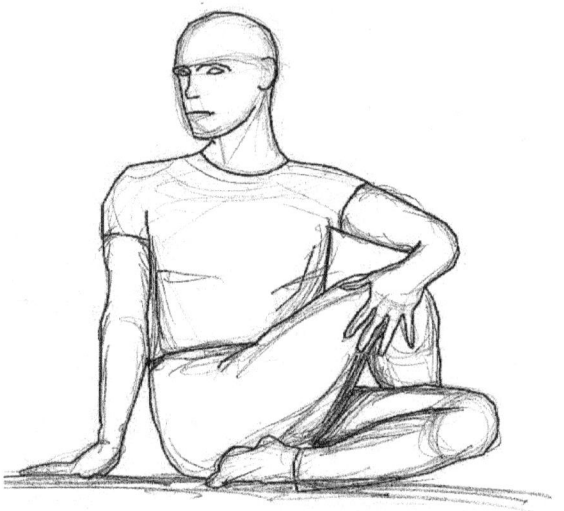

Fig. 59: Spinal Twist

Seated Forward Bend:
- Sit on the floor with your legs straight in front of you.
- Lean forward from the hip joints, not the waist.
- Try to lengthen the front torso into the pose, keeping your head raised.
- Clasp your hands around the ankles and slightly pull into deeper bend.
- Bend the elbows out to the sides.
- Hold for 5 seconds.

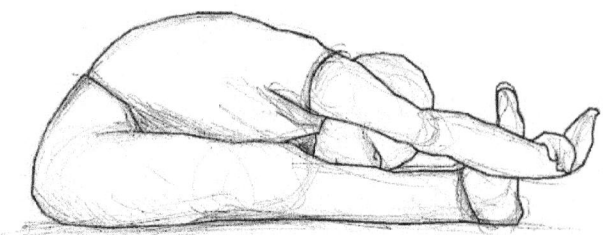

Fig. 60: Forward Bend

Bound Angle Pose

- Sit with your legs out in front of you.
- Exhale, bend your knees and pull your heels toward your center. Put the soles of your feet together.
- Grasp the big toe, or ankle, of each foot. Let your legs open up. Instead of forcing your knees down you can lean forward with your torso. This movement will help open up your hips by gently pushing your knees down.
- Stay in the Angle Pose for 30 seconds.
- Inhale. Extend your legs in front of you.

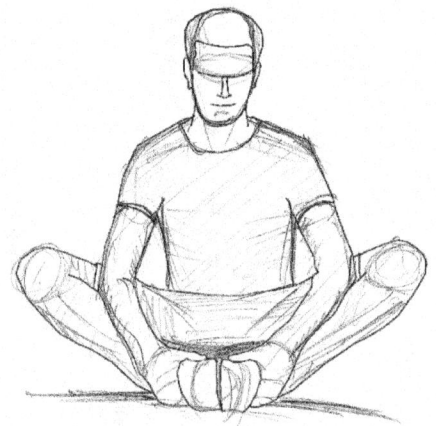

Fig. 61: Bound Angle Pose

Plow Pose

- Lie down on the floor.
- Bring your legs over your head and slowly lower them floor beyond your head.
- Keep your torso perpendicular to the floor and your legs fully extended.
- Press your hands against your back.
- Hold the pose for 10 seconds.
- Start rolling out of the pose.

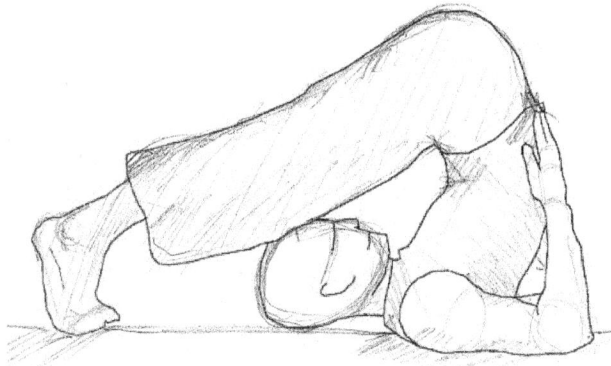

Fig. 62: Plow Pose

Supported Shoulder Stand

- Slowly continue the rolling out motion from previous pose.
- Raise your legs straight up. Lift your lower back up as much as you can (Fig. 57). Keep

your bent arms on your lower back locking your upper body in a supported position. Make sure your body is not bent at your hips.
- When your legs are at your highest point make your final pull at your core (or center, or abdominal).
- Stay in the Shoulder Stand Pose for 10 seconds.
- Slowly lower your legs. Then stop supporting your upper body. Slowly bring your legs over your head and lower (unroll) them to the Corpse Pose.

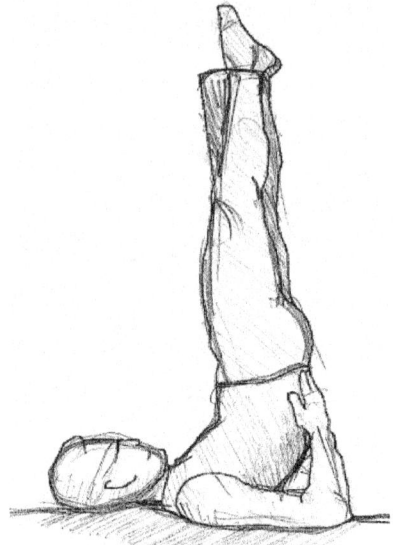

Fig. 63: Shoulder Stand

Rest or Corpse Pose:
- Lie down. Try to get your body into neutral position.
- Extend your arms alongside your body resting backs of the hands on the floor.
- Let shoulder blades rest evenly on the floor.
- Relax all your muscles.
- Stay in this pose 10-20 seconds.

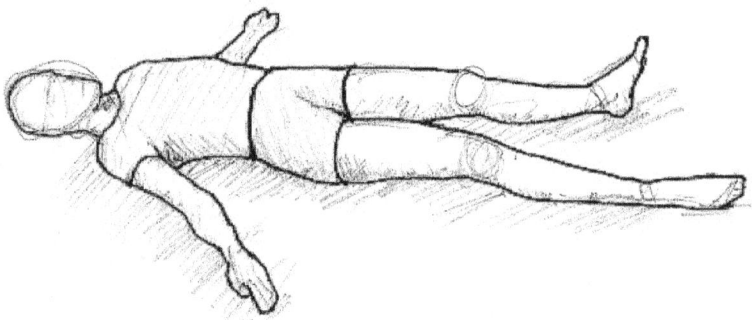

Fig. 64: Corpse Pose

This the end of the routine. It should take you 10 minutes.
Phase 3 checklist can be found at: http://yoga-connect.blogspot.com/

Phase 4

This phase will last 4 months. Unless you have another activity every other day, you can workout 6 days a week. Please take a break on the seventh day. We are adding more exercises including exercises that suppose strengthen your abdominal muscles. This routine takes +/- 18 minutes.

Abdominal Breathing:
- Sit on the mat in a neutral posture and place your hands on the knees.
- Relax your shoulders.
- Inhale. Feel how your abdomen expand like a balloon. Hold for 2 seconds.
- Slowly contract your abdomen by "sucking" in your belly button - exhale.
- Repeat two-three more times.

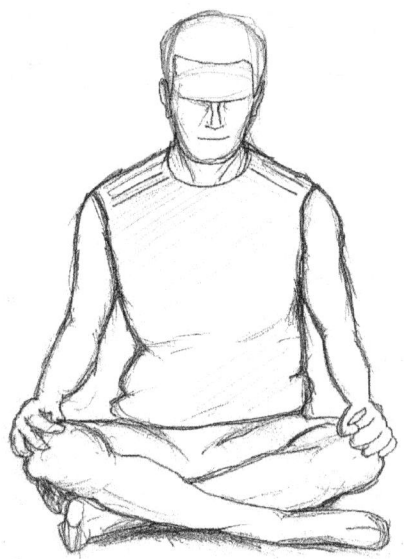

Fig. 65: Neutral Posture

Neck stretching:
- Turn your head up. Look up at the ceiling.
- Turn your head down, "Chin to Chest", look down.
- Repeat, turn your head up.
- Turn your head down.
- Look straight ahead.
- Turn your head 90 degrees to the left.
- Turn back to look straight ahead.
- Turn your head 90 degrees to the right.

- Repeat, turn your head to the left.
- Turn back to look straight ahead.
- Turn your head to the right.
- Look straight ahead. Rest for 2 seconds

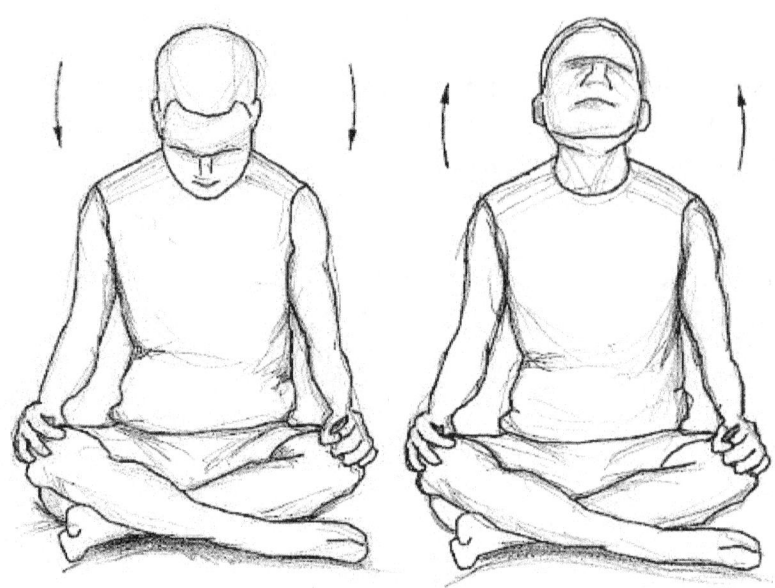

Fig. 66: Head up & down

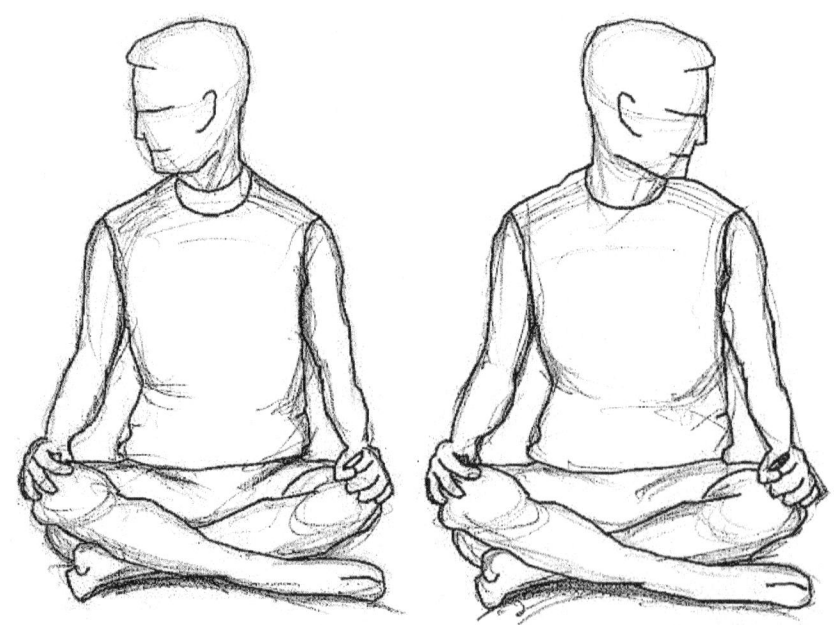

Fig. 67: Head left & right

Neck stretching (continued):

- Gently lower your chin to relax the back of your neck (the only area that is bent is your neck).
- Lower your right ear down towards your shoulder.
- Hold for 2 seconds.
- Return upright.
- Repeat "Ear to Shoulder" on the other side.
- Rest for 2 seconds and repeat the turns two more times.
- Clockwise head rotation – twice.
- Counterclockwise head rotation – twice.

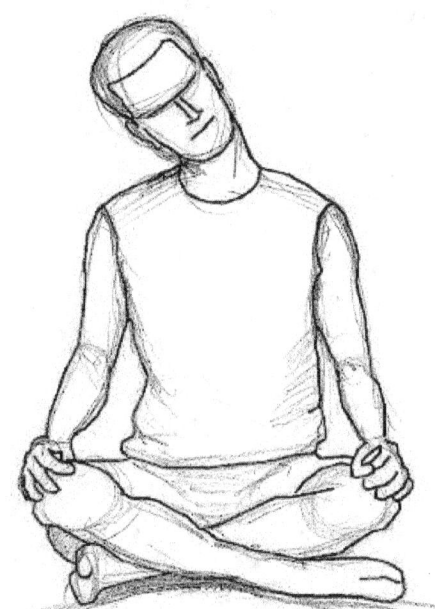

Fig. 68: Ear to Shoulder

Shoulders:

- Shrug your shoulders: while your palms are resting on your knees lift your shoulders and hold for 2 seconds. Let your shoulders drop. Rest for 2 seconds and repeat the shrugs two more times.
- Touch your left ear with your right hand.
- Place your left hand under the elbow of your right hand. Apply pressure on the elbow to force the right hand go far behind your left ear.
- Repeat on the other side.

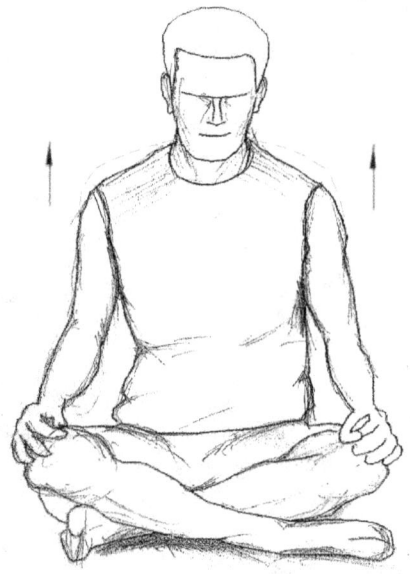

Fig. 69: Shoulder Shrug

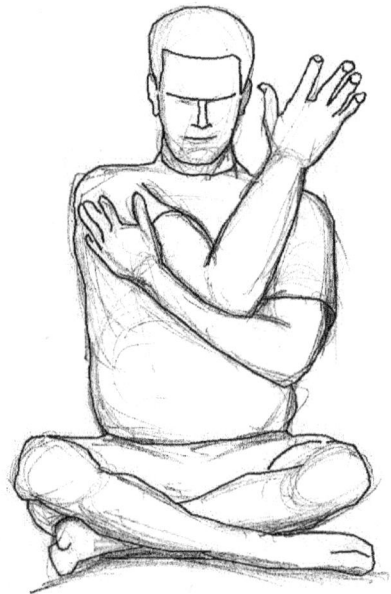

Fig. 70: Shoulder Stretch

Wrist stretch 1
- Put palms of your hands together in front of your chest (as for prayer).
- Pressure your left wrist with your right, slightly bending it back.
- Hold through 2-3 breaths.
- Return to original position.
- Repeat 2 more times

Wrist Stretch 2
- Hold up one hand in front of you like you would when saying "stop."
- Grab your fingers with your other hand and pull your fingers back gently to provide a

stretch to your wrist.
- Relax your shoulders, and hold through four breaths.
- Turn your hand so that your fingers point downward, and the back of your hand faces away from you.
- Take hold of the back of your hand with your other hand and pull gently toward you to stretch the back of your wrist.
- Hold for four breaths.
- Repeat both stretches on the other hand.

Half Back-roll (roll like a ball)
-- If you have any back problems, recent injuries or surgeries, talk to your doctor about this exercise! --

Half Back-roll:

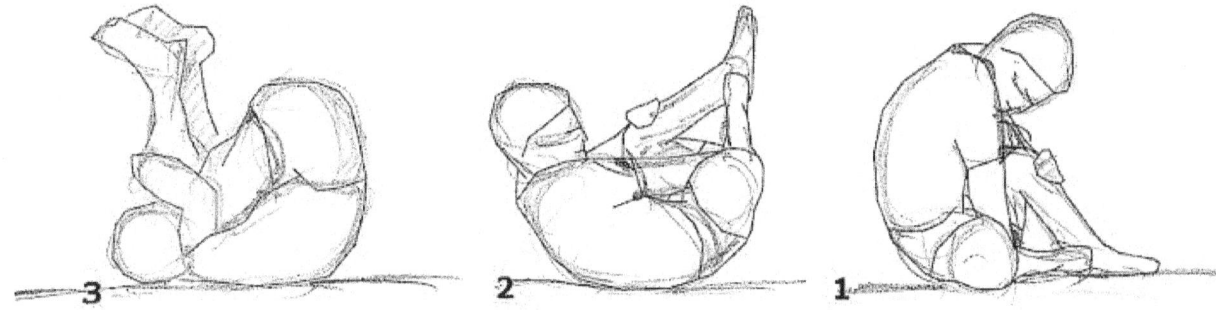

Fig. 71: Back-roll

- Sit on the mat (required – first few times you may use 2 mats) with both legs bent at the knees. One leg is turned so the sides of the thigh and the knee rest on the floor. The knee of the other leg is pointed up and foot is flat on the floor. Keep your chin pressed to your chest.
- Push-off with your front leg and slowly roll on your back.
- When your legs are above your head (and area touching the floor is between your shoulder blades - #3) stop the motion.
- Come back to the original position but switch legs on the way back.
- Stop. Get ready to push-off with the other leg.
- Repeat three (3) more times changing legs on the way back.

Notes:
1. Stop the backward roll when you reach the area between your shoulder blades. While your head and neck will touch the mat they should not get compressed against it.
2. Make your rolling motion smooth.
3. Keep your chin pressed to your chest through out the whole motion.

Sun Salutation A (two sets):
1. Mountain Pose
   Stand straight with big toes touching (heels can be slightly separated). Distribute weight evenly onto four corners of each foot. Firm you muscles. Gently draw in your belly. Pull back your shoulders.
   - Stand in narrow stance with feet parallel to each other, toes touching.
   - Spread your toes.
   - Distribute your weight evenly on your feet. (You can accomplish that by slowly rocking back and forth.) Let your feet "root down" into the floor.
   - Tighten leg muscles.
   - Pull the shoulders back to open your chest.
   - Take several deep breaths.

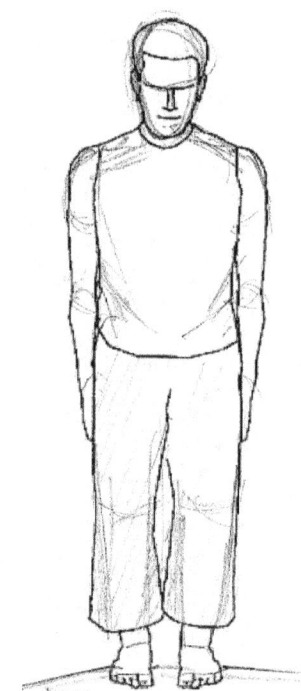

Fig. 72: Mountain Pose

2. Prayer Pose - Exhale
   Stand erect with your feet together, exhale. Keep hands joined together, as if you were praying, in front of your chest. Keep your gaze straight ahead.

3. Raised Arms Pose - Inhale
   Inhaling, while keeping your palms together raise your arm arms up over your head until they are straight, look toward hands.

   When you raise your arms don't just raise them, extend them. Extend them farther. You should feel your shoulders being stretched.

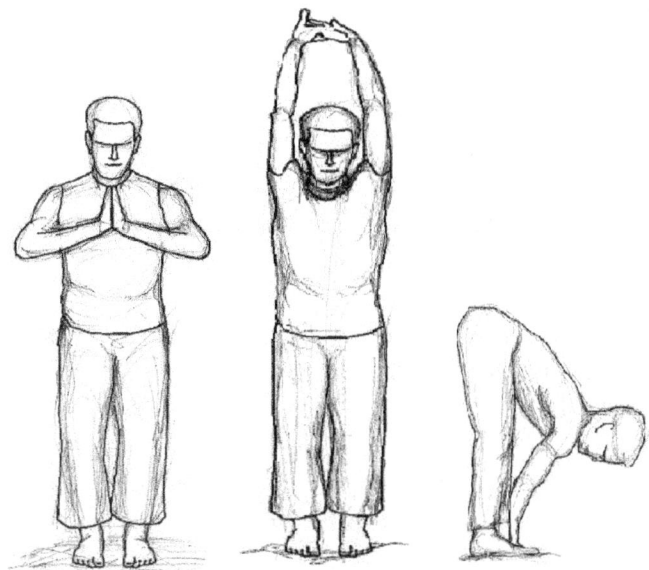

Fig. 73: Prayer - Raised Arms - Half Forward Bend poses

4. Half Forward Bend Pose - Inhale
    Inhaling, straighten your arms, lift the torso so it is parallel to the floor. Extend and straighten your spine. Place your fingertips on the floor. Look toward a wall in front of you.

    The most important thing in this pose is to keep the spine flat. If you can't place your hands on the floor or you can't do that without curving your back use the blocks under your hands.

5. Plank Pose – hold your breath.
    Place palms on the floor just outside of the feet. Step right foot back into lunge, lower hips. Step your left leg back into push-up position (top of push-up). The arms should be straight and perpendicular to the floor. Shoulders directly over the wrists, torso parallel to the floor. The feet should be on the balls. Backs of your legs and torso should form a straight line.

    This pose strengthens your arms. However, there is a variation of this pose, also called plank, where arms are bent at the elbows (forearms rest on the floor) and it works on abdominal muscles.

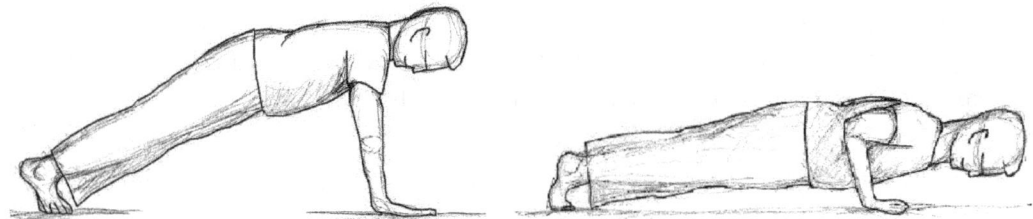

Fig. 74: Plank - Four-Limbed Staff poses

6. Four-Limbed Staff Pose - Exhale
    Exhaling bend elbows and lower body toward floor until it is 2-3 inches above it (lower push-up position). Gaze down. Hold for 10 seconds.

    Unlike in any other pose, in this pose you will feel that you are using your muscles. You will have to control your descent and then hold your body just off the floor. (If you lower your body slowly to the floor it maybe better then 2-3 pushups.)

7. Cobra Pose - Inhale
    Inhaling, roll your feet over the tips of your toes (the feet may also stay on the balls), lower your hips and thighs toward the floor (touch or almost touch the floor), lift your chest on straight arms. Look straight up.

    This pose will strengthen your spine, stretch the chest, shoulders, and abdomen, firm the buttocks, and relieve stress and fatigue.

8. Downward Dog Pose - Exhale
    Exhaling, push the hips up while rolling your feet back over the tips of your toes. Lift your midsection up. Straighten your legs, try to let your heels touch the floor, stretch out your arms so they are in line with your torso. Look at the floor. Hold.

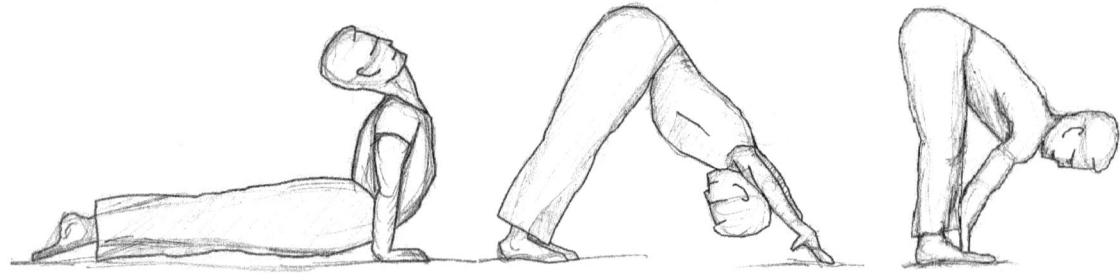

Fig. 75: Cobra - Downward Dog - Half Forward Bend poses

9. Half Forward Bend Pose - Inhale
    Look up between your hands. Inhaling step right foot up between your hands, then step your left foot in next to your right foot. Straighten your arms and legs. The torso should be parallel to the floor. Place your fingertips on the floor. Look straight forward.

10. Forward Bend Pose - Exhale
    While exhaling: lower your torso toward floor keeping the spine straight. Place your fingertips on the floor just outside your feet. The fingertips should be aligned with your toes. Bring the torso and head toward your legs in forward fold.

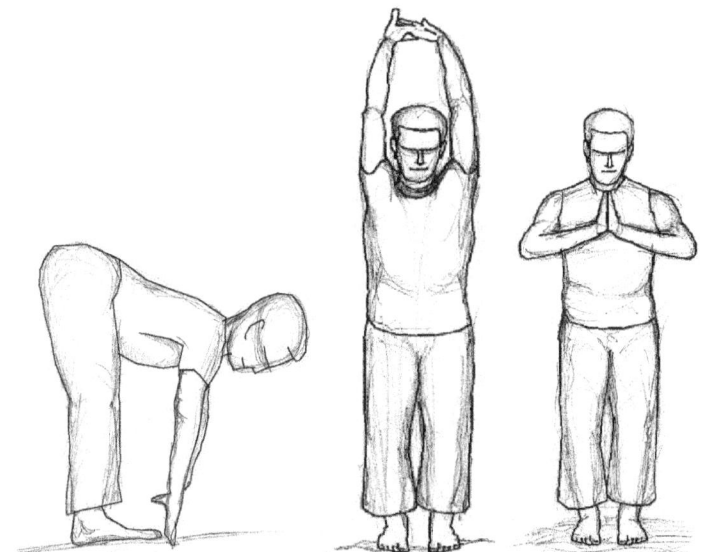

Fig. 76: Forward Bend - Raised Arms – Prayer poses

11. Raised Arms Pose - Inhale
    While inhaling: lift your torso up to the standing position, sweep your arms up overhead, the palms come together.

12. Return to Prayer Pose - Exhale
    Lower the hands in front of your chest to the prayer position.
    Then, release the arms by the sides of your body.

Sun Salutation B (two sets)
Sun Salutation B is a longer sequence of movements then Sun Salutation A. It builds up heat within the body. If you are doing it with intensity, you will break sweat.

1. Prayer Pose - Exhale
   Standing erect with feet together, exhale. Keep hands joined together, as if you were praying, in front of your chest. Keep your gaze straight ahead.

2. Raise your hands over the head – hold your breath.

3. Chair Pose - Inhale
   Inhaling, bend knees, lower hips until thighs are almost parallel to the floor. Sweep arms out and up toward the ceiling, palms face in, bring torso more vertical into Chair pose. This is a deep squat pose. It engages your legs, back, and ankles. If you are a skier you will see its benefits better then anyone.

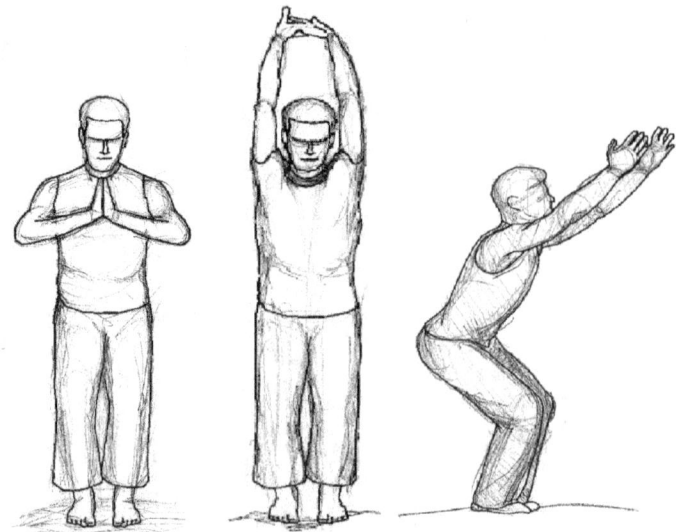

Fig. 77: Prayer - Chair poses

4. Forward Bend Pose – Exhale
    While exhaling: keeping the spine straight lower your torso toward the floor, place your fingertips on the floor just outside your feet, the fingertips should be in line with the toes. Bring the torso and head toward legs in a forward fold. Try to place your hands flat on the floor.

5. Half Forward Bend Pose - Inhale
    Inhaling, straighten your arms, lift the torso so it is parallel to the floor. Extend and straighten your spine. Place your fingertips on the floor. Look toward a wall in front of you. Place palms on the floor just outside of feet (transition). Step right foot back into lunge, lower hips. Step your left leg back into pushup position (top of pushup position). The arms should be perpendicular to the floor. The feet should be on the balls. Backs of your legs and torso should form a straight line.

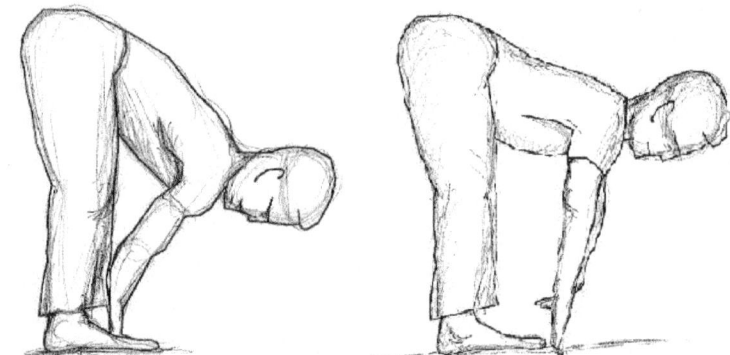

Fig. 78: Forward Bend - Half Forward Bend poses

6. Plank Pose - Transition
    Place palms on the floor just outside of the feet. Step right foot back into lunge, lower hips. Step your left leg back into push-up position (top of push-up). The arms should be perpendicular to the floor. The feet should be on the balls. Backs of your legs and torso should form a straight line.

This pose strengthens your arms. However, there is a variation of this pose, also called plank, were arms are bent at the elbows (forearms rest on the floor) and it works on abdominal muscles.

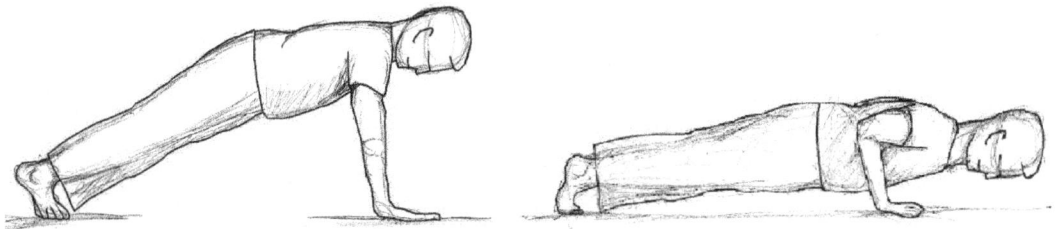

Fig. 79: Plank – Four-Limbed Staff poses

7. Four-Limbed Staff Pose - Exhale
    Exhaling bend elbows and lower body toward floor until you almost touch it (lower push-up position). Gaze down. Hold for 10 seconds.

8. Cobra Pose - Inhale
    Inhaling, roll your feet over the tips of your toes (the feet may also stay on the balls), lower your hips and thighs toward the floor (touch or almost touch the floor), lift your chest on straight arms. Look straight up.

9. Downward Dog Pose - Exhale
    Exhaling, push the hips up while rolling your feet back over the tips of your toes. Lift your midsection up. Straighten your legs, try to let your heels touch the floor, stretch out your arms so they are in line with your torso. Look at the floor. Hold.

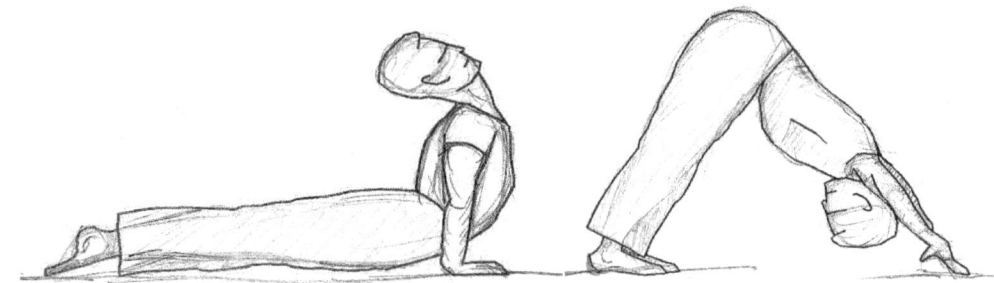

Fig. 80: Cobra - Downward Dog poses

10. Warrior I Pose - Inhale
    While inhaling make a step with your right leg. Raise your hands above the head. Bring palms together. Gaze at the thumbs. Hold for 10 seconds. Slightly bend your knees, step back into Plank.
    The pose strengthens the legs (long step) and opens the chest.

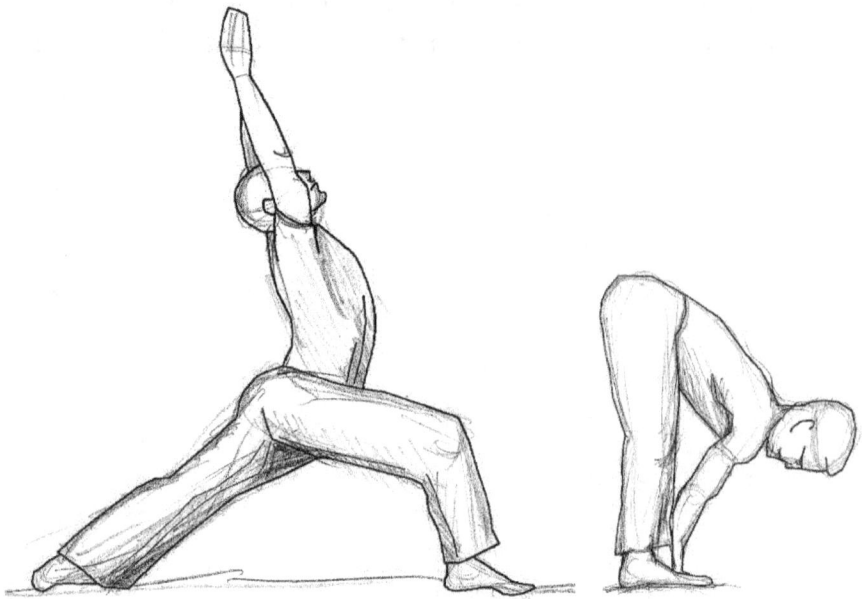

Fig. 81: Warrior I - Forward Bend poses

11. Forward Bend Pose – Exhale
    While exhaling: keeping the spine straight lower your torso toward the floor, place your
    fingertips on the floor just outside your feet, the fingertips should be in line with the toes.
    Bring the torso and head toward legs in a forward fold. Try to place your hands flat on the
    floor.
    This pose can be used as a resting position between the standing poses. Stay in the pose
    for 10 seconds.

12. Half Forward Bend Pose - Inhale
    Inhaling, straighten your arms, lift the torso so it is parallel to the floor. Extend and
    straighten your spine. Place your fingertips on the floor. Look toward a wall in front of
    you. Place palms on the floor just outside of feet (transition). Step right foot back into
    lunge, lower hips. Step your left leg back into pushup position (top of pushup position).
    The arms should be perpendicular to the floor. The feet should be on the balls. Backs of
    your legs and torso should form a straight line

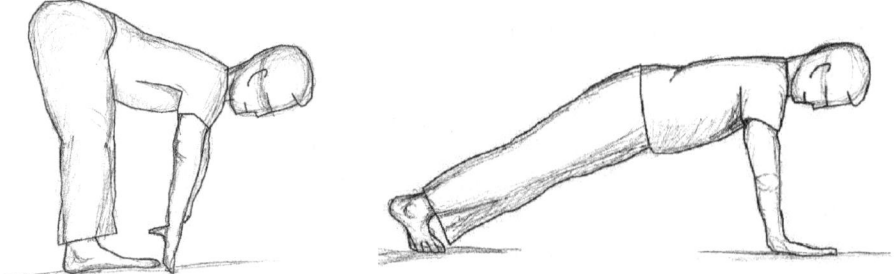

Fig. 82: Half Forward Bend - Plank poses

13. Plank Pose - Transition
    Place palms on the floor just outside of the feet. Step right foot back into lunge, lower
    hips. Step your left leg back into push-up position (top of push-up). The arms should be

perpendicular to the floor. The feet should be on the balls. Backs of your legs and torso should form a straight line.

14. Four-Limbed Staff Pose - Exhale
    Exhaling bend elbows and lower body toward floor almost touching it. Gaze down. Hold for 10 seconds.

15. Cobra Pose - Inhale
    Inhaling, roll your feet over the tips of your toes (the feet may also stay on the balls), lower your hips and thighs toward the floor (touch or almost touch the floor), lift your chest on straight arms. Look straight up.

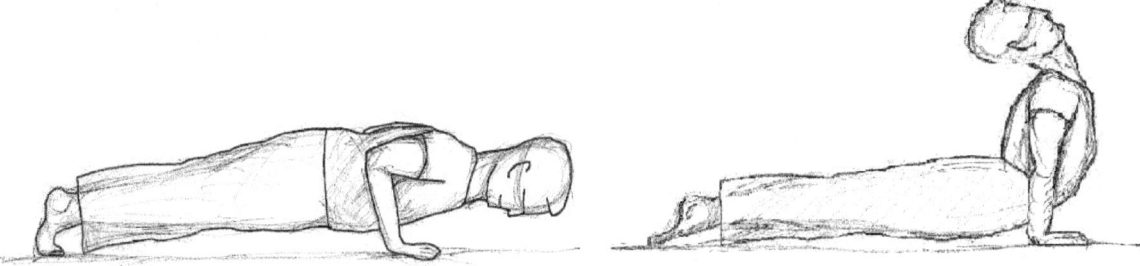

Fig. 83: Four-Limbed Staff – Cobra poses

16. Downward Dog Pose - Exhale
    Exhaling, push the hips up while rolling your feet back over the tips of your toes. Lift your midsection up. Straighten your legs, try to let your heels touch the floor, stretch out your arms so they are in line with your torso. Look at the floor. Hold.

17. Begin inhaling as you look up between hands. Step left foot up between hands.

18. Warrior I Pose - Inhale
    Continue inhaling as you rise into Warrior Pose. Sweep arms overhead. Bring palms together. Gaze at the thumbs.

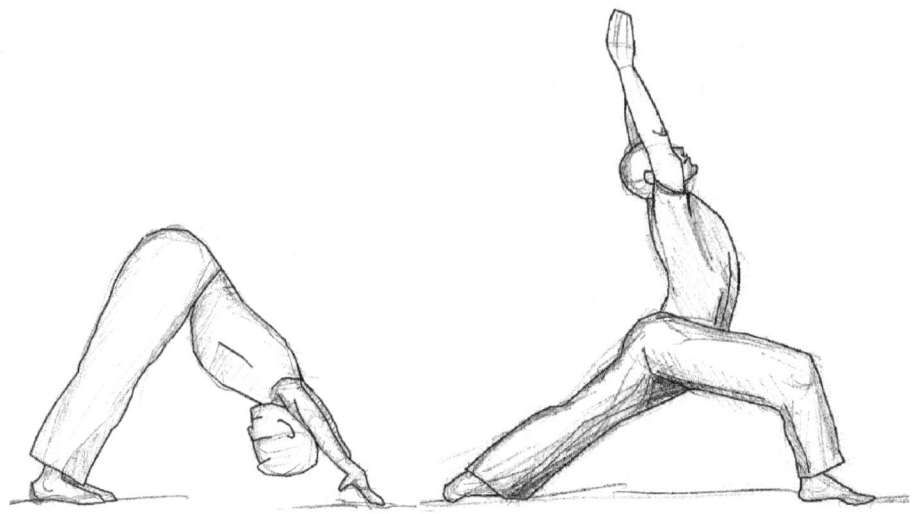

Fig. 84: Downward - Warrior I poses

19. Forward Bend Pose – Exhale
   While exhaling: keeping the spine straight lower your torso toward the floor, place your fingertips on the floor just outside your feet, the fingertips should be in line with the toes. Bring the torso and head toward legs in a forward fold. Try to place your hands flat on the floor.
   Stay in the pose for 30 seconds to 1 minute.

20. Half Forward Bend Pose - Inhale
   Inhaling, straighten your arms, lift the torso so it is parallel to the floor. Extend and straighten your spine. Place your fingertips on the floor. Look toward a wall in front of you. Place palms on the floor just outside of feet (transition). Step right foot back into lunge, lower hips. Step your left leg back into pushup position (top of pushup position). The arms should be perpendicular to the floor. The feet should be on the balls. Backs of your legs and torso should form a straight line.

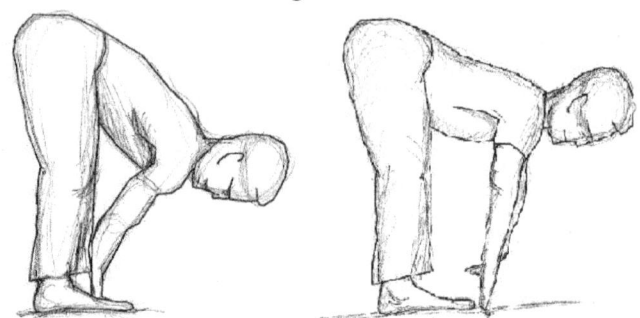

Fig. 85: Forward & Half Forward Bend poses

21. Plank Pose - Transition
   Place palms on the floor just outside of the feet. Step right foot back into lunge, lower hips. Step your left leg back into push-up position (top of push-up). The arms should be perpendicular to the floor. The feet should be on the balls. Backs of your legs and torso should form a straight line.

22. Four-Limbed Staff Pose - Exhale
   Exhaling place palms on the floor. Step back into the Plank Pose. Exhaling bend elbows and lower body toward floor. Gaze down. Hold for 10 seconds.

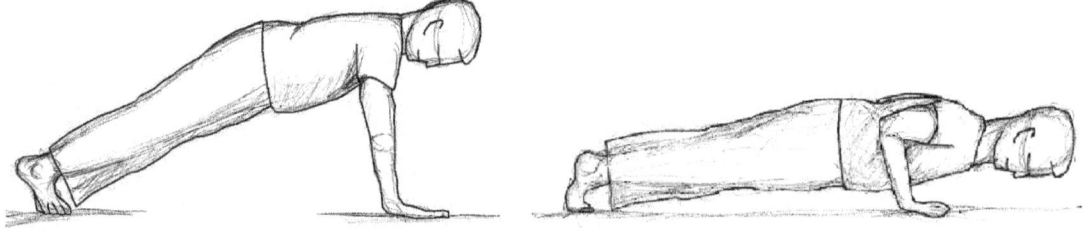

Fig. 86: Plank & Four-Limbed Staff poses

23. Cobra Pose - Inhale
   Inhaling, roll your feet over the tips of your toes (the feet may also stay on the balls), lower your hips and thighs toward the floor (touch or almost touch the floor), lift your chest on straight arms. Look straight up.

24. Downward Dog Pose - Exhale

    Exhaling, push the hips up while rolling your feet back over the tips of your toes. Lift your midsection up. Straighten your legs, try to let your heels touch the floor, stretch out your arms so they are in line with your torso. Look at the floor. Hold.

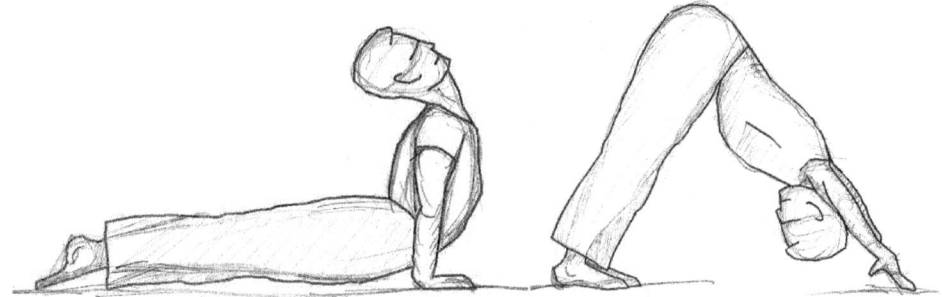

Fig. 87: Cobra & Downward Dog poses

25. Begin inhaling as you look up between hands. Step left foot up between hands.

26. Half Forward Bend Pose - Inhale

    Look up between your hands. Inhaling step right foot up between your hands, then step your left foot in next to your right foot. Straighten your legs and arms. The torso should be parallel to the floor. Place your fingertips on the floor. Look straight forward.

27. Forward Bend Pose - Exhale

    Inhaling, straighten your arms, lift the torso so it is parallel to the floor. Extend and straighten your spine. Place your fingertips on the floor. Look toward a wall in front of you. Bring the torso and head toward your legs in forward fold.

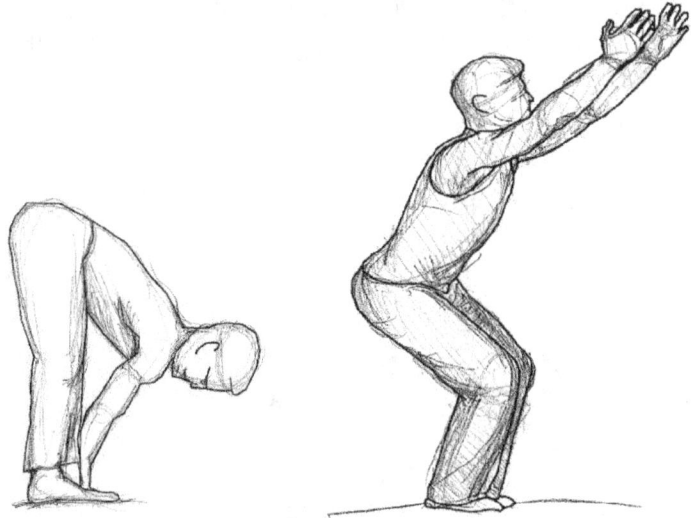

Fig. 88: Forward Ben & Chair poses

28. Chair Pose - Inhale

    Inhaling, bend knees, lower hips until thighs are almost parallel to the floor. Sweep arms out and up toward the ceiling, palms face in, bring torso more vertical into Chair pose.

29. Raised Arms Pose - Hold breath
    While inhaling: lift your torso up to the standing position, sweep your arms up overhead, the palms come together.

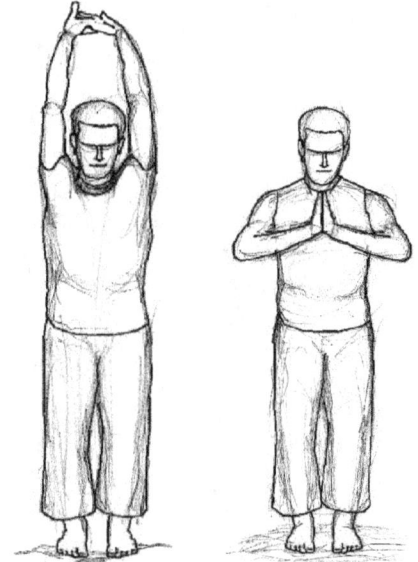

Fig. 89: Raised Arms & Prayer poses

30. Prayer Pose - Exhale

Extended Triangle Pose

Step back left leg about 4ft, keep your legs straight. Toes at front foot should point ahead. Back foot should be perpendicular to the front one (pointing to the side). Extend your arms so they are parallel to the floor, palms turned down. Align back heel to with front heel. Front arm should be directly over front leg, the same side, pointing straight ahead. Back arm should be directly over back leg, pointing back. Bend your torso by lowering your right hand to the right shin or ankle on the inner side of the foot while the left hand points straight up. Stay in it for 10 seconds.

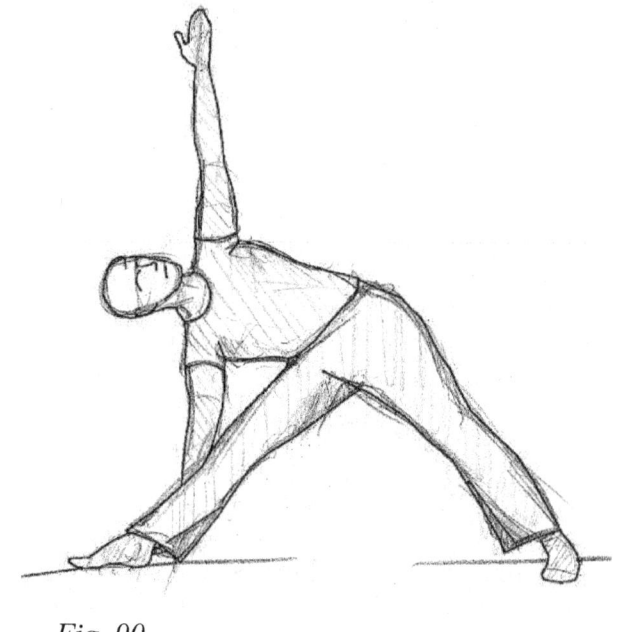

Fig. 90

Come up from the pose, just torso. Switch sides by turning your hips and repeat for the same length of time.

Warrior II Pose
Come up from the previous pose. Switch sides by turning your hips. Keep arms parallel to the floor. Try to reach as far as you can. Both feet turned as they were in the previous pose. Bend your front knee so that the shin is perpendicular to the floor. Look straight ahead. Stay in the pose for 10 seconds. Breathe slowly. Come up from the pose. Repeat on the other side.

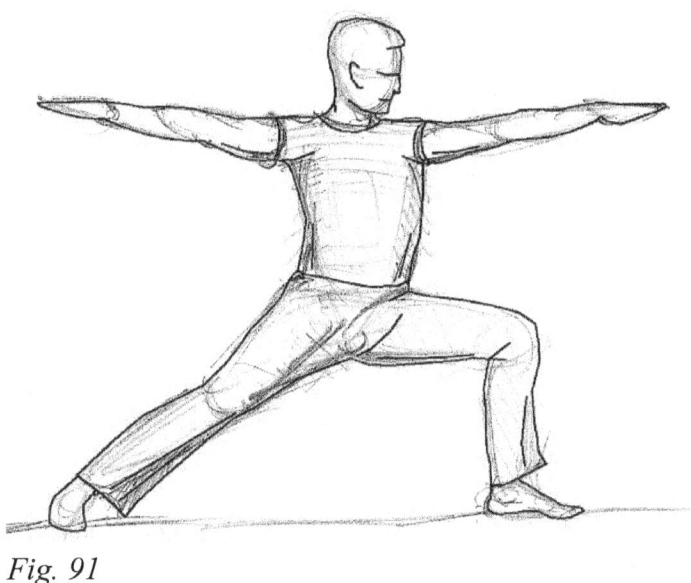

Fig. 91

Wide-Legged Forward Bend
Feet 3 - 4 feet apart parallel to each other. Place hands on your hips. Bend forward as much as you can. Hold 10-15 seconds. Place your hands on the floor and try even deeper bend. This is Wide-Legged Forward Bend. Stay in it for 10 seconds.

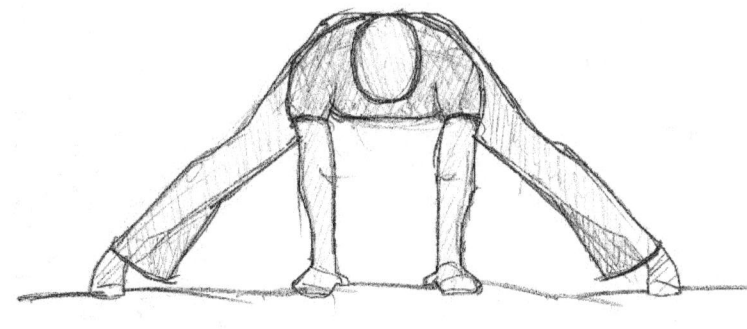

Fig. 92

Tree Pose
- Start with a Mountain Pose.
- Shift your weight onto your left foot, bend your right knee and lift your right foot bringing it to the center.

- Place the sole of your right foot on the inner left thigh. You can start right above the knee. As you are more comfortable, you can progress to the point where you cannot bring your leg any higher.
- Press your palms together in front of your chest and raise them above your head. Look straight ahead.

(If you need to support your pose you can hold your leg with one hand, preferably from the same side, and raise the other hand over your head.)

Stay in the Tree Pose from 10 seconds to 20 seconds. Repeat on the other side.

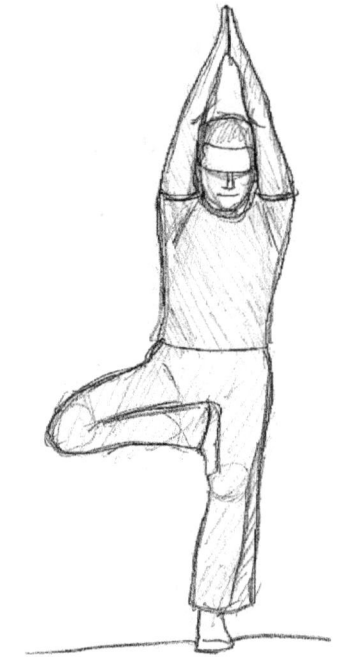

Fig. 93: Tree Pose

Superman Pose
1. Lie face-down on the floor, feet together, chin on the floor.
2. Stretch the arms in front of you as far as you can.
3. Breathing in, raise the upper torso, arms, and legs. Keep your elbows and knees straight.
4. Hold and continue with long, gentle breaths (in and out). Breathing out, release and relax.

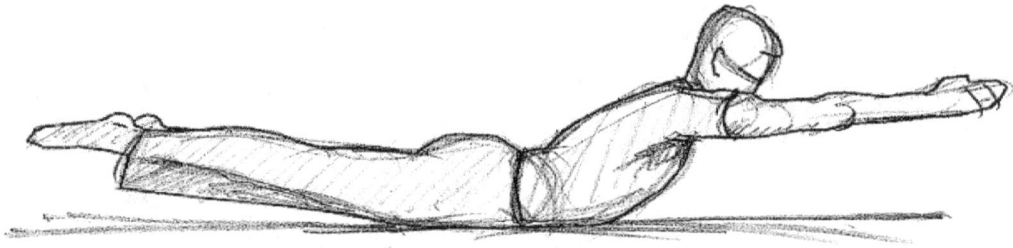

Fig. 94: Superman Pose

Benefits:
Tones the arms and legs. Strengthens abdominal muscles and lower back.

Locust Pose
- Lie on your belly with your arms along the sides of your torso, palms up.
- Rotate your thighs by turning your big toes toward each other. Firm your buttocks.
- Exhale and lift your head, upper torso, arms, and legs away from the floor.
- Raise your arms parallel to the floor and stretch them back through your fingertips.
- Gaze forward or slightly upward.

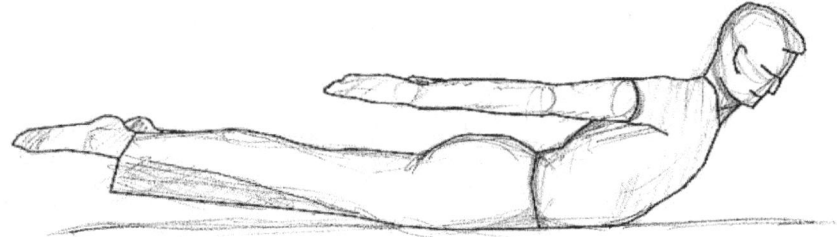

Fig. 95: Locust Pose

Stay in the pose from 10 seconds to 20 seconds, then release with an exhalation. Take a breath and repeat 1 or 2 times.

Bridge Pose
- Lie down on the floor. Arms on the sides.
- Bend your knees and place your feet firmly on the floor as close to your buttocks as possible.
- Lift your hips off the floor. Keep your arms flat on the floor. Your feet and thighs should be parallel, 4 - 6 inches apart. Lift your hips as much as you can. The knees should be directly over the heels. Your spine should arch so you much that only top your shoulder, neck and back of your head touch the floor.

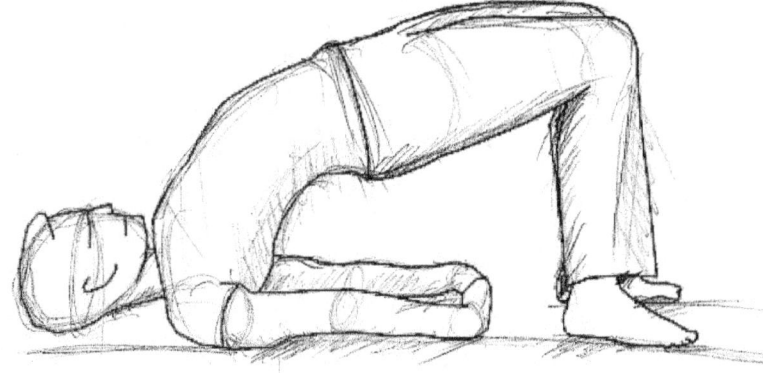

Fig. 96: Bridge Pose

Stay in the Bridge Pose for 10 seconds or little more. When you release from the pose roll the spine down slowly onto the floor.

Half Boat Pose
- Lie supine on the mat.
- Lift your legs 6 inches above the floor.
- Lift your upper body 6 inches above the floor with hands along the body. Hold for 30 seconds. Both legs and upper body are only a half the distance from the floor, hence… Half Boat Pose. Hold it for 10 seconds.

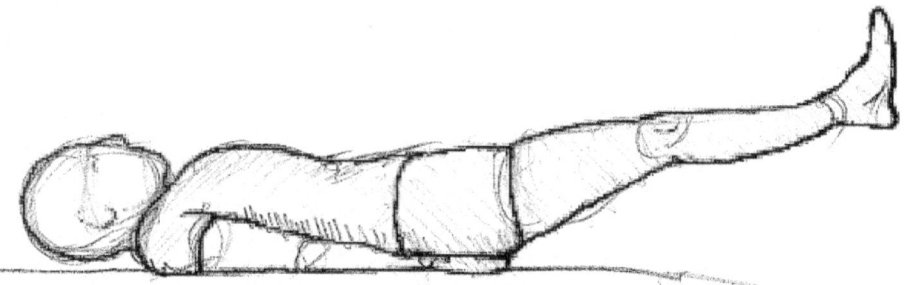

Fig. 97: Half Boat Pose

Full Boat Pose
Sit on the floor with your legs in front of you. Knees can be lightly bent. Lean back slightly and extend your arms in front of you. Lift your legs and straighten them so they are plus/minus 45 degrees from the floor.

If you ever "google" this pose and look at the images the search returns, you will see that there are many ways to get to this pose. Each one is correct. The differences are the result of differences in our bodies and how we accomplish the balance.

Because the balance is not that easy, your pose may look differently every time you try.

Stay in the Full Boat Pose from 10 seconds to 1 minute.

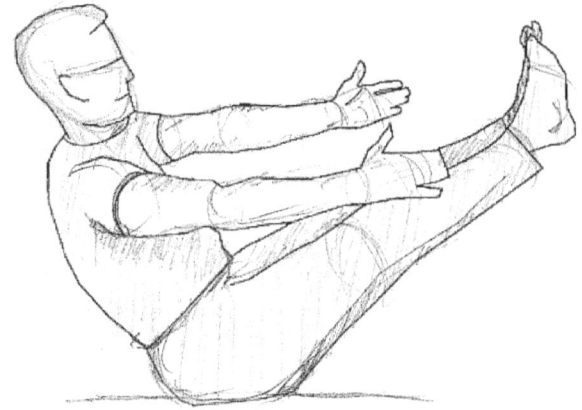

Fig. 98: Full Boat

Head to the Knee:
- Sit with straight legs in front of you.

- Pull the left leg to the center and place the foot sole lightly against the inner thigh of the right leg so the shin is at a right angle to the right leg.
- While holding the left ankle with the left hand grab the right ankle with the other hand. Pull your head to the right knee. Hold for 5-10 seconds.
- Repeat on other side.

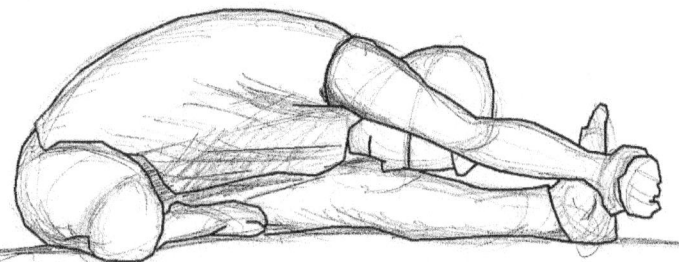

Fig. 99: Head to knee

Spinal Twist:
- Sit with straight legs in front of you.
- Pull the left leg to the center and place the foot under the right leg almost to the buttock.
- Bend the right leg at the knee and place the foot on the floor outside your left thigh. The right knee should point straight up.
- Twist your upper body so that your left shoulder points at the right knee and right shoulder point to the back.
- Place your left hand on the outside thigh of the right leg trying to grab the leg as low as possible.
- The right arm either supports your body. This is the Half Spinal Twist. Stay in it for 5 seconds.
- Repeat on other side.

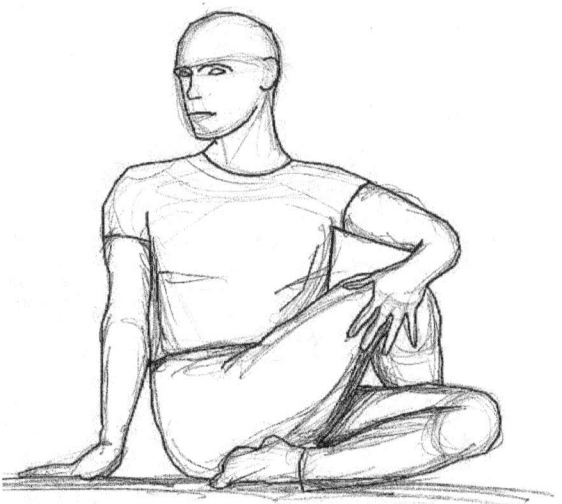

Fig. 100: Spinal Twist

Seated Forward Bend:
- Sit on the floor with your legs straight in front of you.
- Lean forward from the hip joints, not the waist.

- Try to lengthen the front torso into the pose, keeping your head raised.
- Clasp your hands around the ankles and slightly pull into deeper bend.
- Bend the elbows out to the sides.
- Hold for 5 seconds.

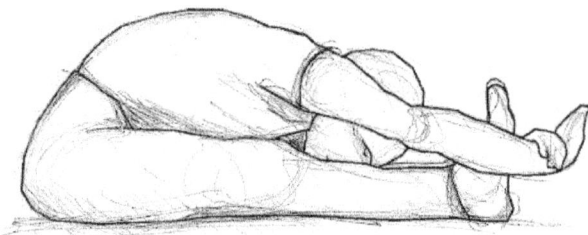

Fig. 101: Forward Bend

Bound Angle Pose
- Sit with your legs out in front of you.
- Exhale, bend your knees and pull your heels toward your center. Put the soles of your feet together.
- Grasp the big toe, or ankle, of each foot. Let your legs open up. Instead of forcing your knees down you can lean forward with your torso. This movement will help open up your hips by gently pushing your knees down.
- Stay in the Angle Pose for 30 seconds.
- Inhale. Extend your legs in front of you.

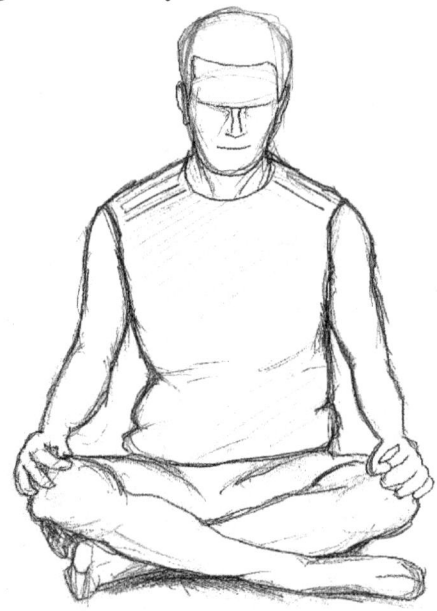

Fig. 102: Bound Angle Pose

Plow Pose
- Lie down on the floor.
- Bring your legs over your head and slowly lower them floor beyond your head.
- Keep your torso perpendicular to the floor and your legs fully extended.
- Press your hands against your back.
- Hold the pose for 10 seconds.

- Start rolling out of the pose.

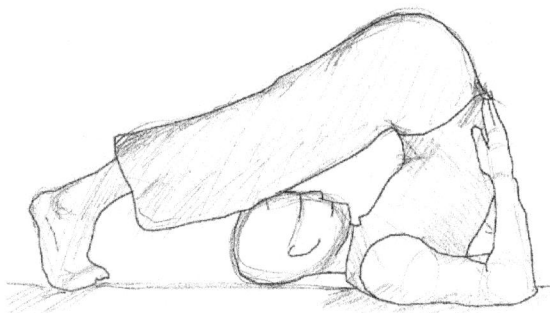

Fig. 103: Plow Pose

Supported Shoulder Stand
- Slowly continue the rolling out motion from previous pose.
- Raise your legs straight up. Lift your lower back up as much as you can (Fig. 57). Keep your bent arms on your lower back locking your upper body in a supported position. Make sure your body is not bent at your hips.
- When your legs are at your highest point make your final pull at your core (or center, or abdominal).
- Stay in the Shoulder Stand Pose for 10 seconds.
- Slowly lower your legs. Then stop supporting your upper body. Slowly bring your legs over your head and lower (unroll) them to the Corpse Pose.

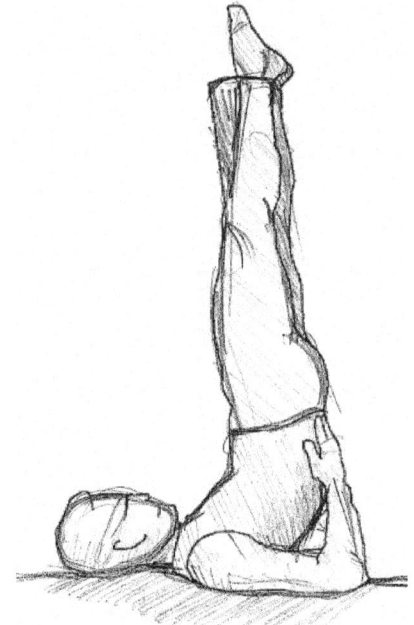

Fig. 104: Shoulder Stand

Rest or Corpse Pose:
- Lie down. Try to get your body into neutral position.
- Extend your arms alongside your body resting backs of the hands on the floor.
- Let shoulder blades rest evenly on the floor.
- Relax all your muscles.

- Stay in this pose 10-20 seconds.

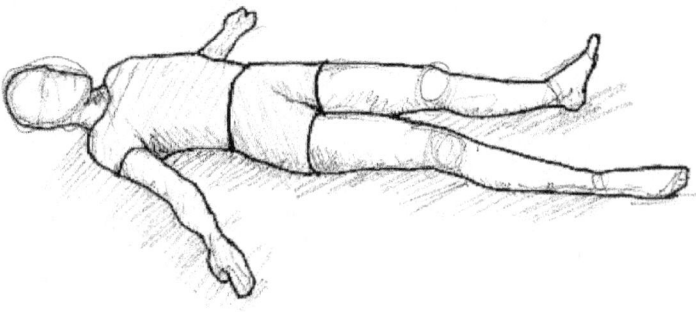

Fig. 105: Corpse Pose

Phase 4 checklist can be found at: http://yoga-connect.blogspot.com/

Phase 5

This phase will last 5 months. If you worked out every day please go back to 3-day a week schedule. On every other day, if you don't have any other sport activity, take a 10-20 minute walk while being mindful of your breathing. Keep it steady. Again, take a break on the seventh day. We are adding more exercises including exercises that suppose strengthen your abdominal muscles. This routine takes +/- 25 minutes. Some of the poses repeat themselves in this phase. The reason for that is simple. We are not trying to go by a list of poses that need to be done, but we are following a sequence of movements. They are in a natural flow. Some poses require counter poses. Other are a logical next step.

Abdominal Breathing:
- Sit on the mat in a neutral posture and place your hands on the knees.
- Relax your shoulders.
- Inhale. Feel how your abdomen expand like a balloon. Hold for 2 seconds.
- Slowly contract your abdomen by "sucking" in your belly button - exhale.
- Repeat two-three more times.

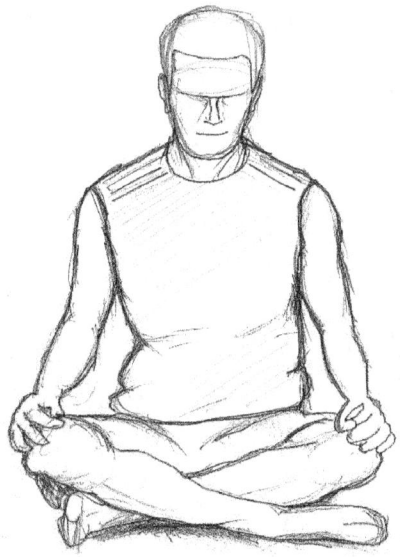

Fig. 106: Neutral Posture

Neck stretching:
- Turn your head up. Look up at the ceiling.
- Turn your head down, "Chin to Chest", look down.
- Repeat, turn your head up.
- Turn your head down.
- Look straight ahead.

- Turn your head 90 degrees to the left.
- Turn back to look straight ahead.
- Turn your head 90 degrees to the right.
- Repeat, turn your head to the left.
- Turn back to look straight ahead.
- Turn your head to the right.
- Look straight ahead. Rest for 2 seconds

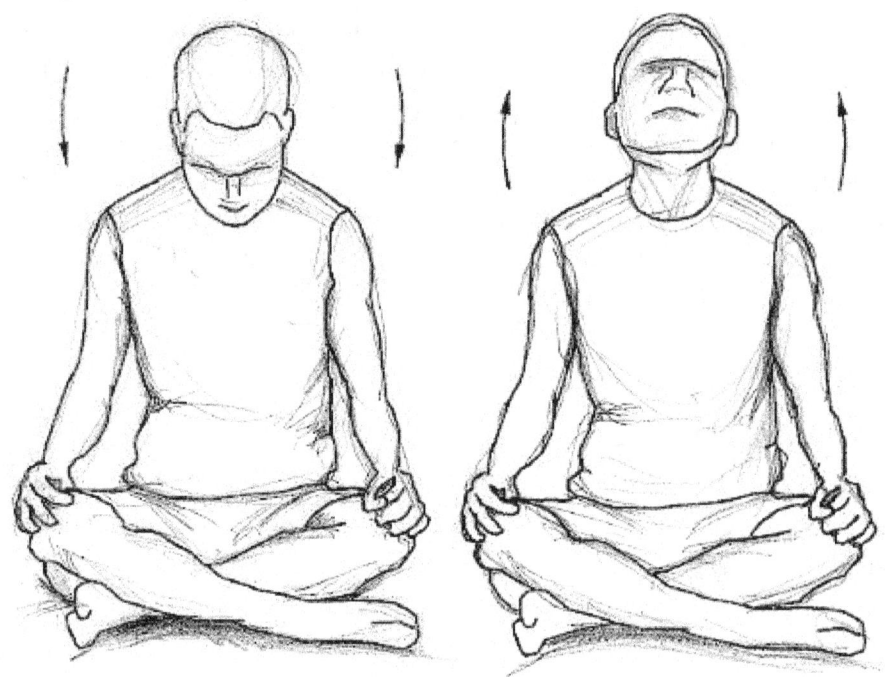

Fig. 107: Head up & down

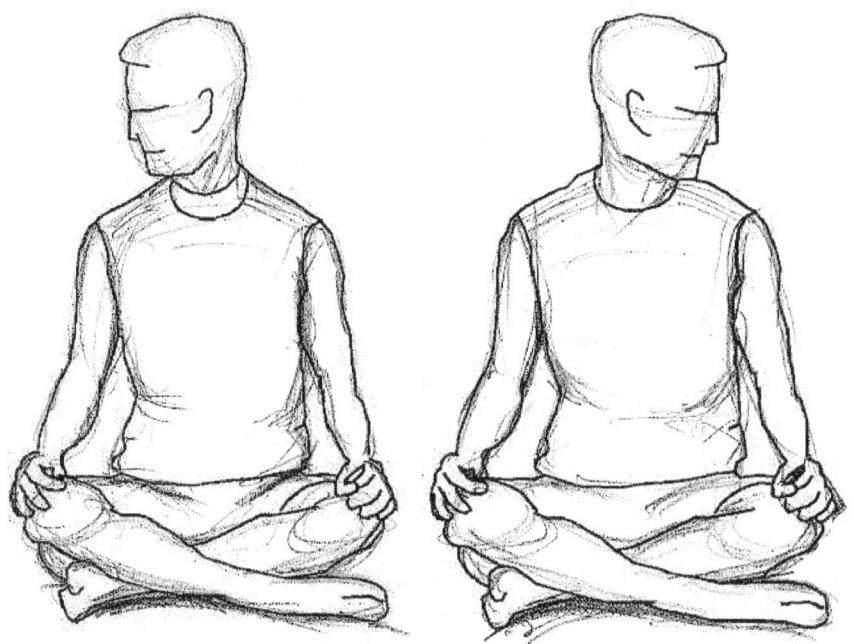

Fig. 108: Head left & right

Neck stretching (continued):
- Gently lower your chin to relax the back of your neck (the only area that is bent is your neck).
- Lower your right ear down towards your shoulder.
- Hold for 2 seconds.
- Return upright.
- Repeat "Ear to Shoulder" on the other side.
- Rest for 2 seconds and repeat the turns two more times.
- Clockwise head rotation – twice.
- Counterclockwise head rotation – twice.

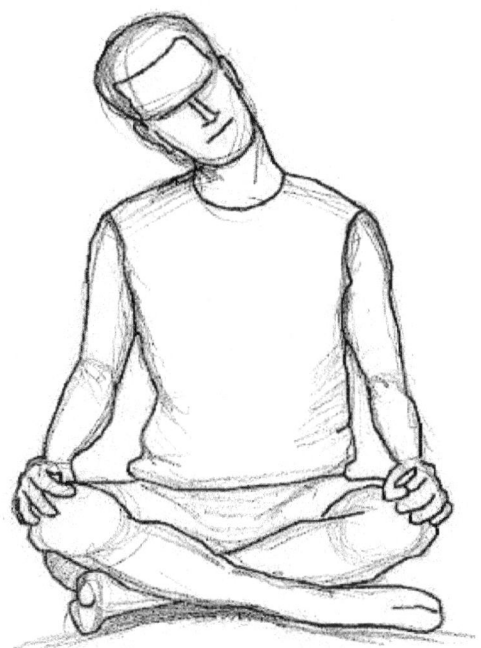

Fig. 109: Ear to Shoulder

Shoulders:
- Shrug your shoulders: while your palms are resting on your knees lift your shoulders and hold for 2 seconds. Let your shoulders drop. Rest for 2 seconds and repeat the shrugs two more times.
- Touch your left ear with your right hand.
- Place your left hand under the elbow of your right hand. Apply pressure on the elbow to force the right hand go far behind your left ear.
- Repeat on the other side.

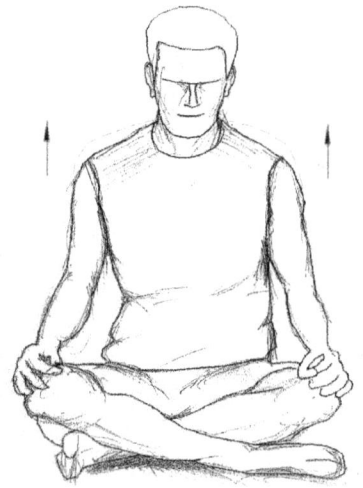

Fig. 110: Shoulder Shrug

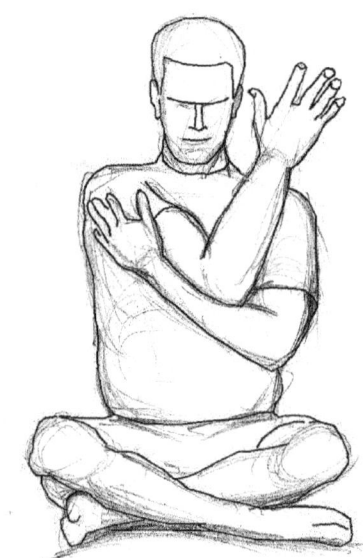

Fig. 111: Shoulder Stretch

Wrist stretch 1
- Put palms of your hands together in front of your chest (as for prayer).
- Pressure your left wrist with your right, slightly bending it back.
- Hold through 2-3 breaths.
- Return to original position.
- Repeat 2 more times

Wrist Stretch 2
- Hold up one hand in front of you like you would when saying "stop."
- Grab your fingers with your other hand and pull your fingers back gently to provide a stretch to your wrist.
- Relax your shoulders, and hold through four breaths.
- Turn your hand so that your fingers point downward, and the back of your hand faces

away from you.
- Take hold of the back of your hand with your other hand and pull gently toward you to stretch the back of your wrist.
- Hold for four breaths.
- Repeat both stretches on the other hand.

Half Back-roll (roll like a ball)
-- If you have any back problems, recent injuries or surgeries, talk to your doctor about this exercise! --

Half Back-roll:

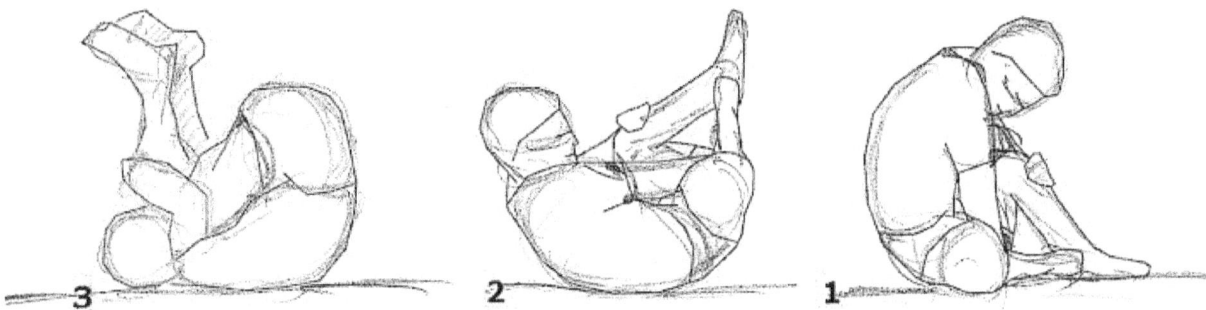

Fig. 112: Back-roll

- Sit on the mat (required – first few times you may use 2 mats) with both legs bent at the knees. One leg is turned so the sides of the thigh and the knee rest on the floor. The knee of the other leg is pointed up and foot is flat on the floor. Keep your chin pressed to your chest.
- Push-off with your front leg and slowly roll on your back.
- When your legs are above your head (and area touching the floor is between your shoulder blades - #3) stop the motion.
- Come back to the original position but switch legs on the way back.
- Stop. Get ready to push-off with the other leg.
- Repeat three (3) more times changing legs on the way back.

Notes:
1. Stop the backward roll when you reach the area between your shoulder blades. While your head and neck will touch the mat they should not get compressed against it.
2. Make your rolling motion smooth.
3. Keep your chin pressed to your chest through out the whole motion.

Sun Salutation A (2 or 4 sets):
1. Mountain Pose
   Stand straight with big toes touching (heels can be slightly separated). Distribute weight

evenly onto four corners of each foot. Firm you muscles. Gently draw in your belly. Pull back your shoulders.

- Stand in narrow stance with feet parallel to each other, toes touching.
- Spread your toes.
- Distribute your weight evenly on your feet. (You can accomplish that by slowly rocking back and forth.) Let your feet "root down" into the floor.
- Tighten leg muscles.
- Pull the shoulders back to open your chest.
- Take several deep breaths.

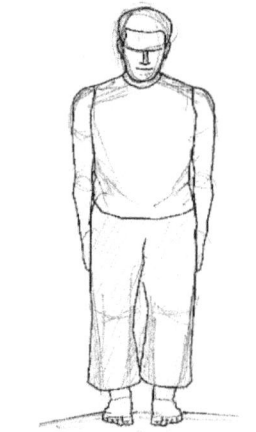

Fig. 113: Mountain Pose

2. Prayer Pose - Exhale
   Stand erect with your feet together, exhale. Keep hands joined together, as if you were praying, in front of your chest. Keep your gaze straight ahead.

3. Raised Arms Pose - Inhale
   Inhaling, while keeping your palms together raise your arm arms up over your head until they are straight, look toward hands.

   When you raise your arms don't just raise them, extend them. Extend them farther. You should feel your shoulders being stretched.

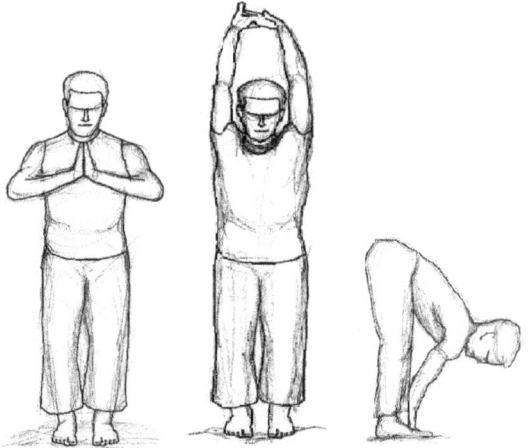

Fig. 114: Prayer - Raised Arms - Half Forward Bend poses

4. Half Forward Bend Pose - Inhale
    Inhaling, straighten your arms, lift the torso so it is para llel to the floor. Extend and straighten your spine. Place your fingertips on the floor. Look toward a wall in front of you.

    The most important thing in this pose is to keep the spine flat. If you can't place your hands on the floor or you can't do that without curving your back use the blocks under your hands.

5. Plank Pose – hold your breath.
    Place palms on the floor just outside of the feet. Step right foot back into lunge, lower hips. Step your left leg back into push-up position (top of push-up). The arms should be straight and perpendicular to the floor. Shoulders directly over the wrists, torso parallel to the floor. The feet should be on the balls. Backs of your legs and torso should form a straight line.

    This pose strengthens your arms. However, there is a variation of this pose, also called plank, where arms are bent at the elbows (forearms rest on the floor) and it works on abdominal muscles.

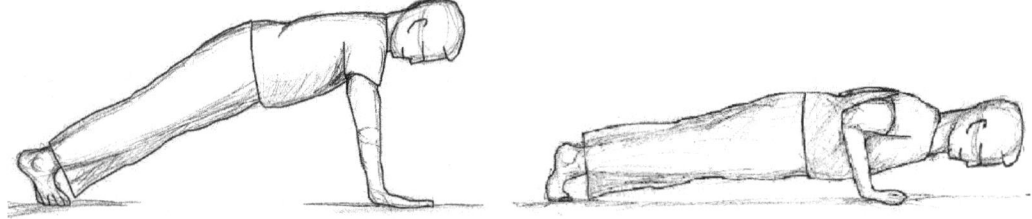

Fig. 115: Plank - Four-Limbed Staff poses

6. Four-Limbed Staff Pose - Exhale
    Exhaling bend elbows and lower body toward floor until it is 2-3 inches above it (lower push-up position). Gaze down. Hold for 10 seconds.

    Unlike in any other pose, in this pose you will feel that you are using your muscles. You will have to control your descent and then hold your body just off the floor. (If you lower your body slowly to the floor it maybe better then 2-3 pushups.)

7. Cobra Pose - Inhale
    Inhaling, roll your feet over the tips of your toes (the feet may also stay on the balls), lower your hips and thighs toward the floor (touch or almost touch the floor), lift your chest on straight arms. Look straight up.

    This pose will strengthen your spine, stretch the chest, shoulders, and abdomen, firm the buttocks, and relieve stress and fatigue.

8. Downward Dog Pose (Adho Mukha Svanasana) - Exhale
    Exhaling, push the hips up while rolling your feet back over the tips of your toes. Lift your midsection up. Straighten your legs, try to let your heels touch the floor, stretch out your arms so they are in line with your torso. Look at the floor. Hold.

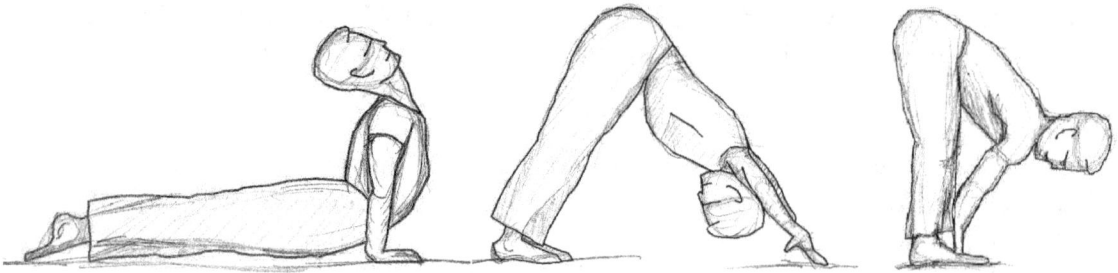

Fig. 116: Cobra - Downward Dog - Half Forward Bend poses

9. Half Forward Bend Pose - Inhale
    Look up between your hands. Inhaling step right foot up between your hands, then step
    your left foot in next to your right foot. Straighten your arms and legs. The torso should
    be parallel to the floor. Place your fingertips on the floor. Look straight forward.

10. Forward Bend Pose - Exhale
    While exhaling: lower your torso toward floor keeping the spine straight. Place your
    fingertips on the floor just outside your feet. The fingertips should be aligned with your
    toes. Bring the torso and head toward your legs in forward fold.

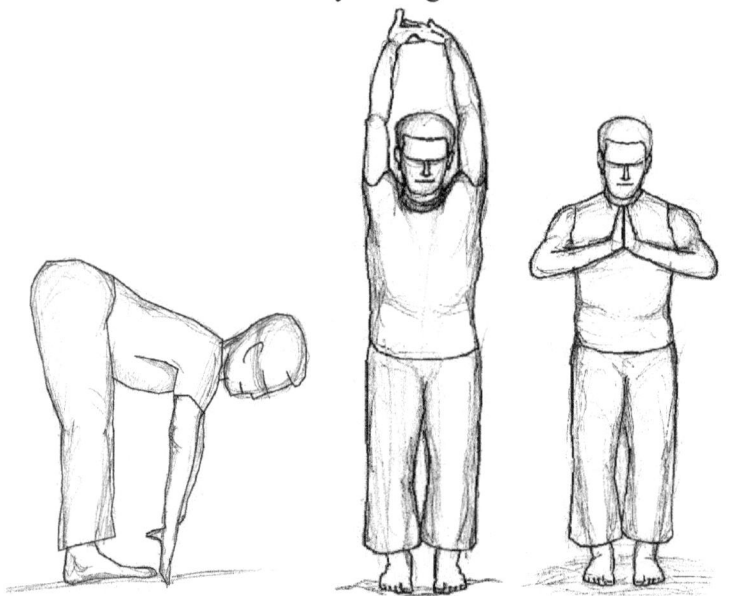

Fig. 117: Forward Bend - Raised Arms – Prayer poses

11. Raised Arms Pose - Inhale
    While inhaling: lift your torso up to the standing position, sweep your arms up overhead,
    the palms come together.

12. Return to Prayer Pose - Exhale
    Lower the hands in front of your chest to the prayer position.
    Then, release the arms by the sides of your body.

Sun Salutation B (2 or 4 sets)
Sun Salutation B is a longer sequence of movements then Sun Salutation A. It builds up heat within the body. If you are doing it with intensity, you will break sweat.

1. Prayer Pose - Exhale
   Standing erect with feet together, exhale. Keep hands joined together, as if you were praying, in front of your chest. Keep your gaze straight ahead.

2. Raise your hands over the head – hold your breath.

3. Chair Pose - Inhale
   Inhaling, bend knees, lower hips until thighs are almost parallel to the floor. Sweep arms out and up toward the ceiling, palms face in, bring torso more vertical into Chair pose. This is a deep squad pose. It engages your legs, back, and ankles. If you are a skier you will see its benefits better then anyone.

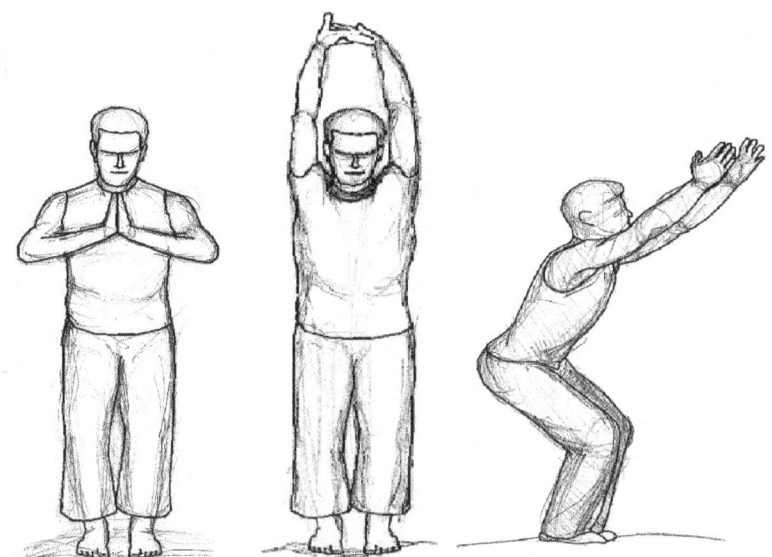

Fig. 118: Prayer - Chair poses

4. Forward Bend Pose – Exhale
   While exhaling: keeping the spine straight lower your torso toward the floor, place your fingertips on the floor just outside your feet, the fingertips should be in line with the toes. Bring the torso and head toward legs in a forward fold. Try to place your hands flat on the floor.

5. Half Forward Bend Pose - Inhale
   Inhaling, straighten your arms, lift the torso so it is parallel to the floor. Extend and straighten your spine. Place your fingertips on the floor. Look toward a wall in front of you. Place palms on the floor just outside of feet (transition). Step right foot back into lunge, lower hips. Step your left leg back into pushup position (top of pushup position). The arms should be perpendicular to the floor. The feet should be on the balls. Backs of your legs and torso should form a straight line.

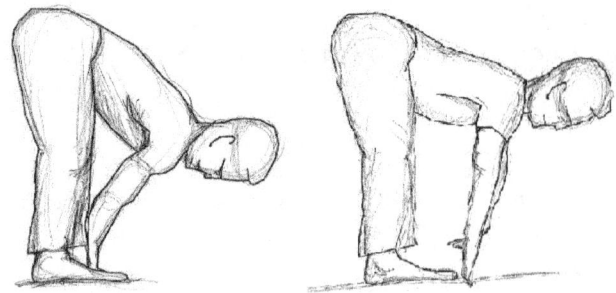

Fig. 119: Forward Bend - Half Forward Bend poses

6. Plank Pose - Transition
    Place palms on the floor just outside of the feet. Step right foot back into lunge, lower hips. Step your left leg back into push-up position (top of push-up). The arms should be perpendicular to the floor. The feet should be on the balls. Backs of your legs and torso should form a straight line.

    This pose strengthens your arms. However, there is a variation of this pose, also called plank, were arms are bent at the elbows (forearms rest on the floor) and it works on abdominal muscles.

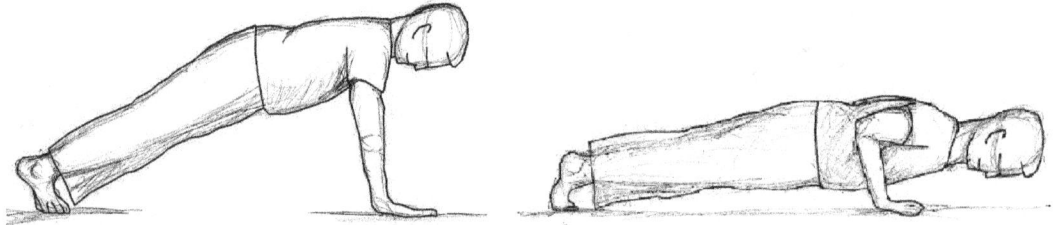

Fig. 120: Plank - Four-Limbed Staff poses

7. Four-Limbed Staff Pose - Exhale
    Exhaling bend elbows and lower body toward floor until you almost touch it (lower push-up position). Gaze down. Hold for 10 seconds.

8. Cobra Pose - Inhale
    Inhaling, roll your feet over the tips of your toes (the feet may also stay on the balls), lower your hips and thighs toward the floor (touch or almost touch the floor), lift your chest on straight arms. Look straight up.

9. Downward Dog Pose - Exhale
    Exhaling, push the hips up while rolling your feet back over the tips of your toes. Lift your midsection up. Straighten your legs, try to let your heels touch the floor, stretch out your arms so they are in line with your torso. Look at the floor. Hold.

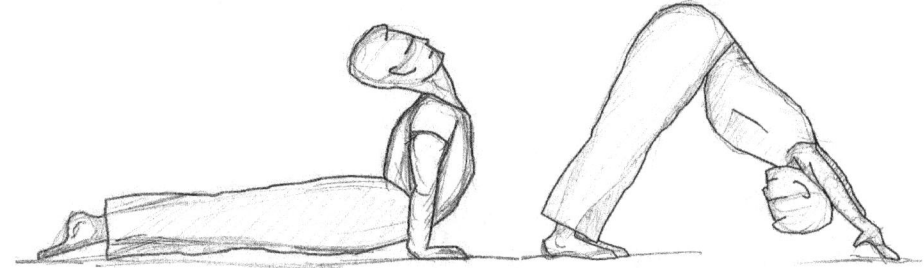

Fig. 121: Cobra - Downward Dog poses

10. Warrior I Pose - Inhale
    While inhaling make a step with your right leg. Raise your hands above the head. Bring palms together. Gaze at the thumbs. Hold for 10 seconds. Slightly bend your knees, step back into Plank.
    The pose strengthens the legs (long step) and opens the chest.

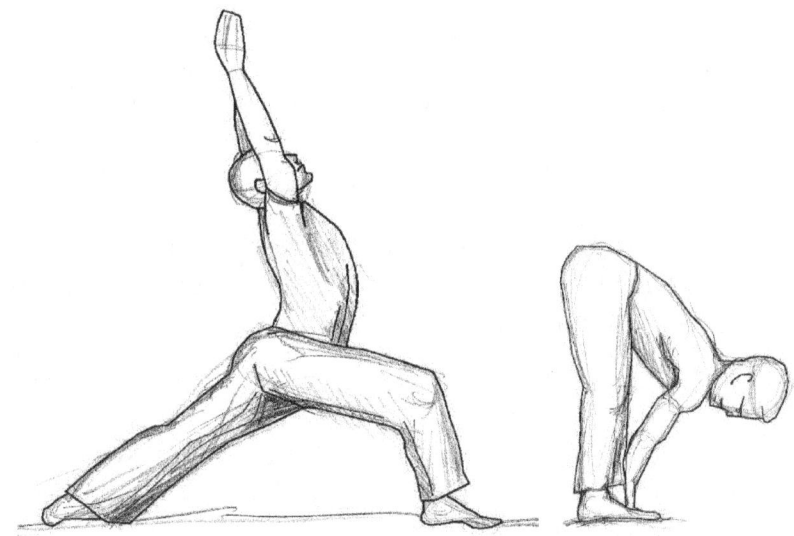

Fig. 122: Warrior I - Forward Bend poses

11. Forward Bend Pose – Exhale
    While exhaling: keeping the spine straight lower your torso toward the floor, place your fingertips on the floor just outside your feet, the fingertips should be in line with the toes. Bring the torso and head toward legs in a forward fold. Try to place your hands flat on the floor.
    This pose can be used as a resting position between the standing poses. Stay in the pose for 10 seconds.

12. Half Forward Bend Pose (Ardha Uttanasana) - Inhale
    Inhaling, straighten your arms, lift the torso so it is parallel to the floor. Extend and straighten your spine. Place your fingertips on the floor. Look toward a wall in front of you. Place palms on the floor just outside of feet (transition). Step right foot back into lunge, lower hips. Step your left leg back into pushup position (top of pushup position). The arms should be perpendicular to the floor. The feet should be on the balls. Backs of your legs and torso should form a straight line.

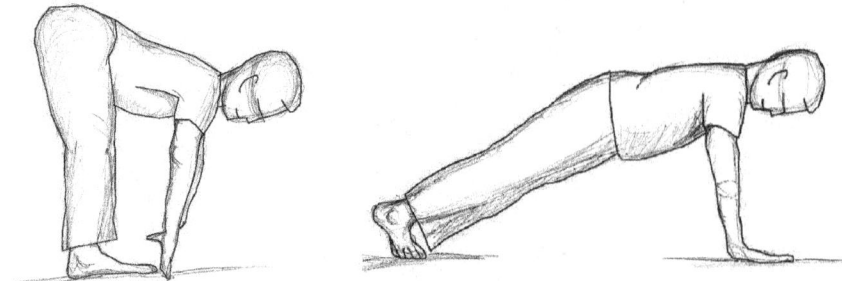

Fig. 123: Half Forward Bend - Plank poses

13. Plank Pose - Transition

    Place palms on the floor just outside of the feet. Step right foot back into lunge, lower hips. Step your left leg back into push-up position (top of push-up). The arms should be perpendicular to the floor. The feet should be on the balls. Backs of your legs and torso should form a straight line.

14. Four-Limbed Staff Pose - Exhale

    Exhaling bend elbows and lower body toward floor almost touching it. Gaze down. Hold for 10 seconds.

15. Cobra Pose - Inhale

    Inhaling, roll your feet over the tips of your toes (the feet may also stay on the balls), lower your hips and thighs toward the floor (touch or almost touch the floor), lift your chest on straight arms. Look straight up.

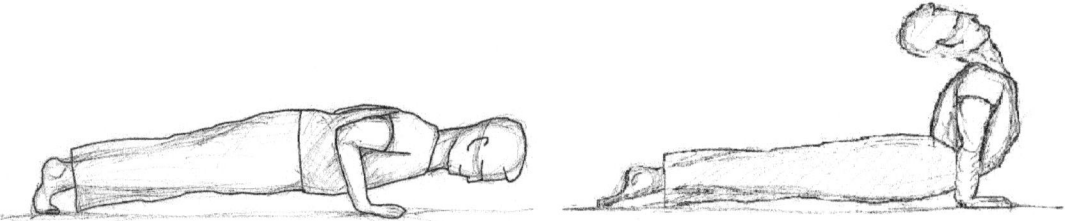

Fig. 124: Four-Limbed Staff – Cobra poses

16. Downward Dog Pose - Exhale

    Exhaling, push the hips up while rolling your feet back over the tips of your toes. Lift your midsection up. Straighten your legs, try to let your heels touch the floor, stretch out your arms so they are in line with your torso. Look at the floor. Hold.

17. Begin inhaling as you look up between hands. Step left foot up between hands.

18. Warrior I Pose - Inhale

    Continue inhaling as you rise into Warrior Pose. Sweep arms overhead. Bring palms together. Gaze at the thumbs.

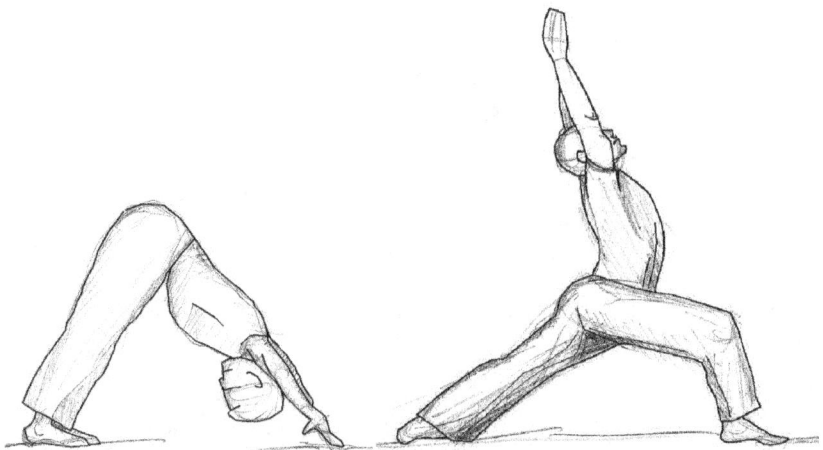

Fig. 125: Downward - Warrior I poses

19. Forward Bend Pose – Exhale
    While exhaling: keeping the spine straight lower your torso toward the floor, place your fingertips on the floor just outside your feet, the fingertips should be in line with the toes. Bring the torso and head toward legs in a forward fold. Try to place your hands flat on the floor.
    This pose can be used as a resting position between the standing poses. Stay in the pose for 30 seconds to 1 minute.

20. Half Forward Bend Pose - Inhale
    Inhaling, straighten your arms, lift the torso so it is parallel to the floor. Extend and straighten your spine. Place your fingertips on the floor. Look toward a wall in front of you. Place palms on the floor just outside of feet (transition). Step right foot back into lunge, lower hips. Step your left leg back into pushup position (top of pushup position). The arms should be perpendicular to the floor. The feet should be on the balls. Backs of your legs and torso should form a straight line.

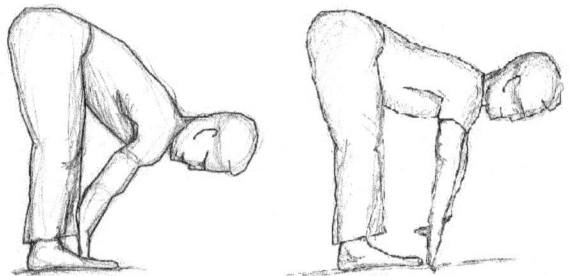

Fig. 126: Forward & Half Forward Bend poses

21. Plank Pose - Transition
    Place palms on the floor just outside of the feet. Step right foot back into lunge, lower hips. Step your left leg back into push-up position (top of push-up). The arms should be perpendicular to the floor. The feet should be on the balls. Backs of your legs and torso should form a straight line.

22. Four-Limbed Staff Pose - Exhale
    Exhaling place palms on the floor. Step back into the Plank Pose. Exhaling bend elbows and lower body toward floor. Gaze down. Hold for 10 seconds.

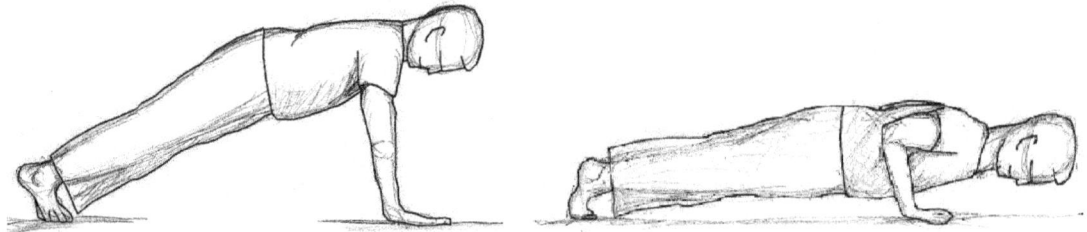

Fig. 127: Plank & Four-Limbed Staff poses

23. Cobra Pose - Inhale
    Inhaling, roll your feet over the tips of your toes (the feet may also stay on the balls), lower your hips and thighs toward the floor (touch or almost touch the floor), lift your chest on straight arms. Look straight up.

24. Downward Dog Pose - Exhale
    Exhaling, push the hips up while rolling your feet back over the tips of your toes. Lift your midsection up. Straighten your legs, try to let your heels touch the floor, stretch out your arms so they are in line with your torso. Look at the floor. Hold.

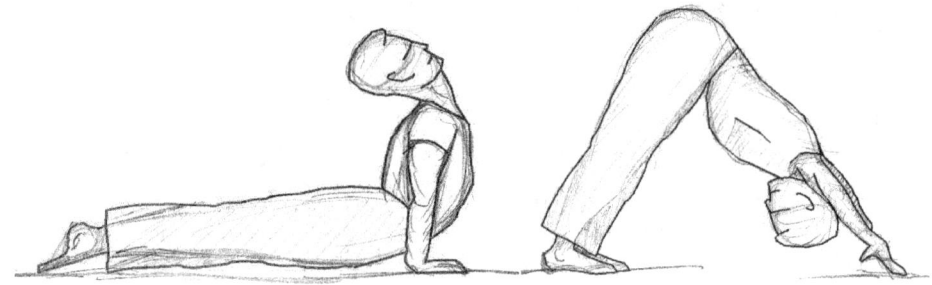

Fig. 128: Cobra & Downward Dog poses

25. Begin inhaling as you look up between hands. Step left foot up between hands.

26. Half Forward Bend Pose - Inhale
    Look up between your hands. Inhaling step right foot up between your hands, then step your left foot in next to your right foot. Straighten your legs and arms. The torso should be parallel to the floor. Place your fingertips on the floor. Look straight forward.

27. Forward Bend Pose - Exhale
    Inhaling, straighten your arms, lift the torso so it is parallel to the floor. Extend and straighten your spine. Place your fingertips on the floor. Look toward a wall in front of you. Bring the torso and head toward your legs in forward fold.

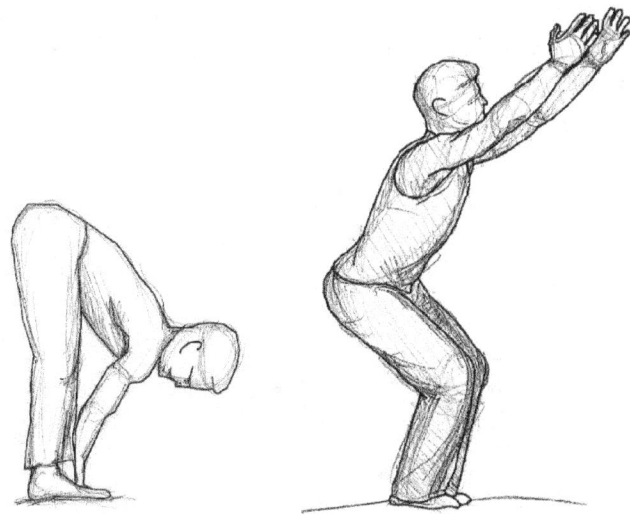

Fig. 129: Forward Bend & Chair poses

28. Chair Pose - Inhale

Inhaling, bend knees, lower hips until thighs are almost parallel to the floor. Sweep arms out and up toward the ceiling, palms face in, bring torso more vertical into Chair pose.

29. Raised Arms Pose - Hold breath

While inhaling: lift your torso up to the standing position, sweep your arms up overhead, the palms come together.

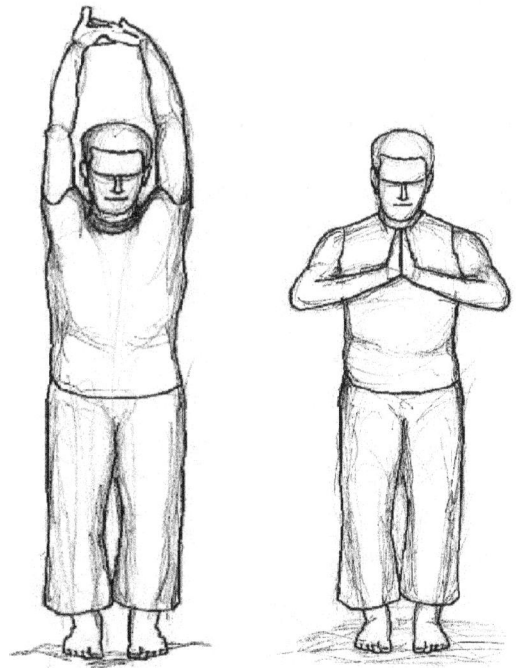

Fig. 130: Raised Arms & Prayer poses

30. Prayer Pose - Exhale

Extended Triangle Pose

Step back left leg about 4ft, keep your legs straight. Toes at front foot should point ahead. Back foot should be perpendicular to the front one (pointing to the side). Extend your arms so they are parallel to the floor, palms turned down. Align back heel to with front heel. Front arm should be directly over front leg, the same side, pointing straight ahead. Back arm should be directly over back leg, pointing back. Bend your torso by lowering your right hand to the right shin or ankle on the inner side of the foot while the left hand points straight up. Stay in it for 10 seconds.

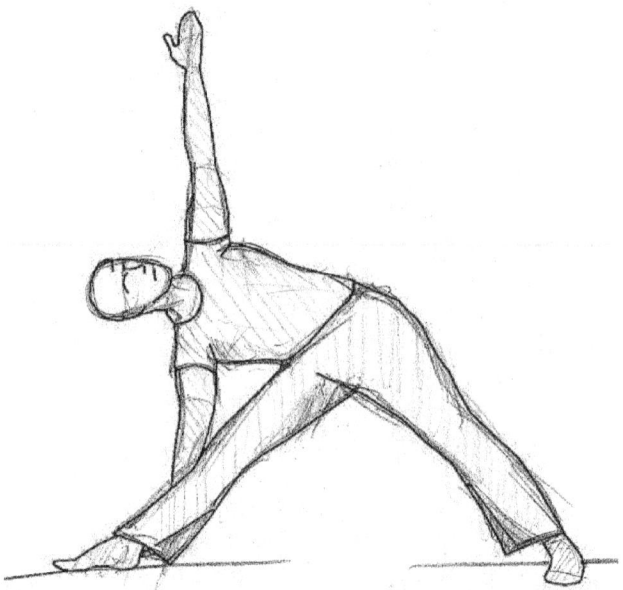

Fig. 131: Extended Triangle Pose

Come up from the pose, just torso. Switch sides by turning your hips and repeat for the same length of time.

Warrior II Pose

Come up from the previous pose. Switch sides by turning your hips. Keep arms parallel to the floor. Try to reach as far as you can. Both feet turned as they were in the previous pose. Bend your front knee so that the shin is perpendicular to the floor. Look straight ahead. This is the Warrior II Pose. Stay in it for 30 seconds. Breathe slowly. Come up from the pose. Repeat on the other side.

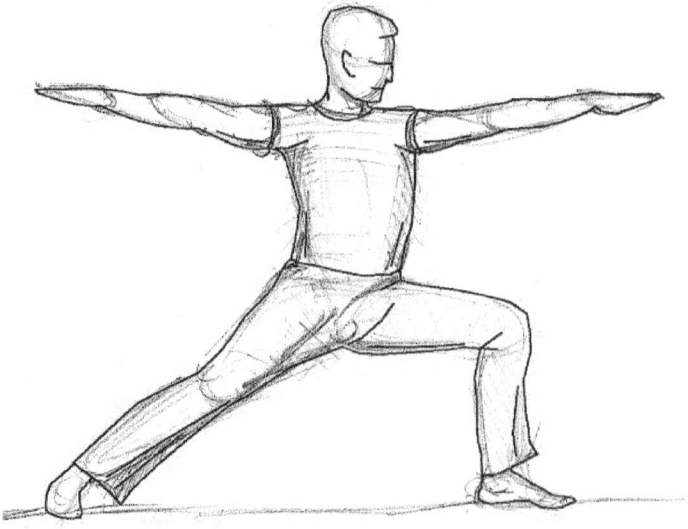

Fig. 132: Warrior II Pose

Extended Side Angle Pose

Switch the sides in the Warrior Pose. Bring the right elbow to the right knee. While you inhale, bring your left arm up and continue the swing so it ends up over your ear. The whole left side of the body should be in a straight line. Stay in it for 10 seconds.

Come up from the pose. Repeat on the other side.

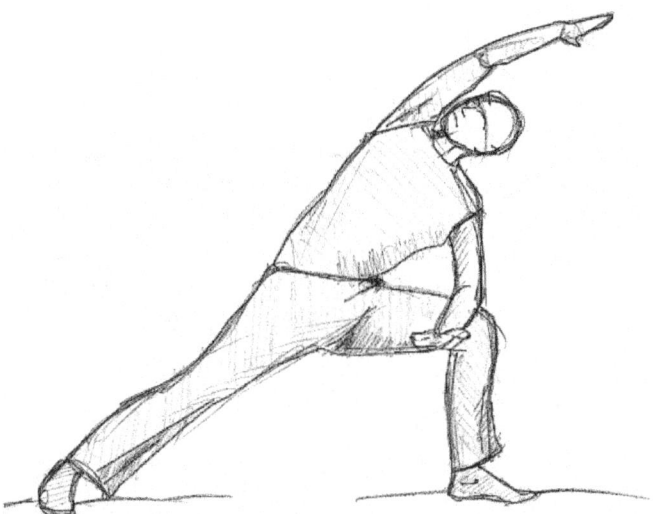

Fig. 133: Extended Side Angle Pose

Warrior I Pose

Come up from the pose. Switch the sides. Again bend your knee just like in previous pose. Clasp your hands together and raise them above your head. Extend your hands strongly. This is the Warrior I Pose. Stay in it for 10 seconds.

Come up from the pose. Repeat on the other side.

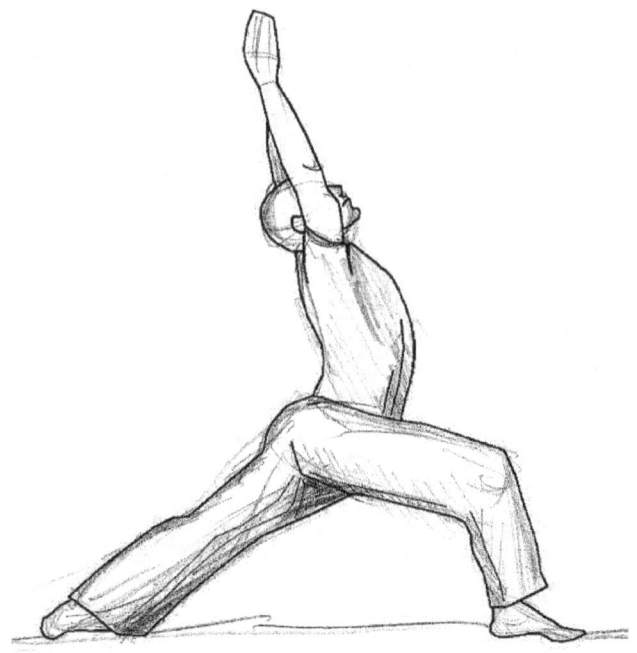

Fig. 134: Warrior 1

Revolving Triangle Pose

Come up from the pose. Switch the sides. Keep both knees straight. Extend your arms so they are parallel to the floor, palms turned down. Align back heel to with front heel. Front arm should be directly over front leg, the same side, pointing straight ahead. Back arm should be directly over back leg, pointing back. Bend and twist your torso by reaching with your back arm to the front ankle (on the outside) and touching the floor with the tips of your fingers. Stay in the pose for 10 seconds.

Come up from the pose. Repeat on the other side.

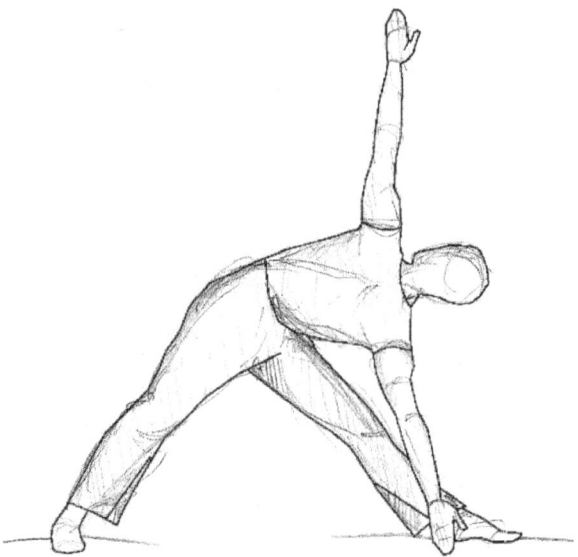

Fig. 135: Revolvving Triangle

Wide-Legged Forward Bend

Feet 3 - 4 feet apart parallel to each other. Place hands on your hips. Bend forward as much as you can. Hold 10-15 seconds. Place your hands on the floor and try even deeper bend. This is Wide-Legged Forward Bend. Stay in it for 30 seconds.

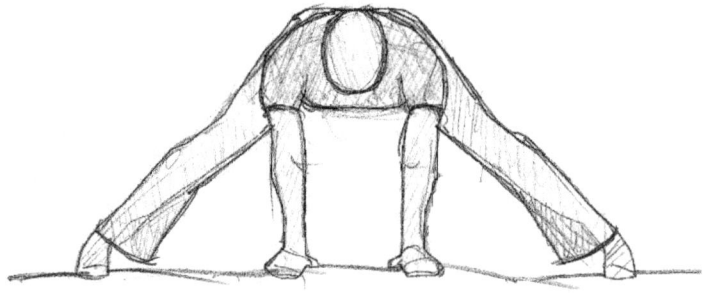

Fig. 136: Wide-Legged Forward Bend

Tree Pose

- Start with a Mountain Pose.
- Shift your weight onto your left foot, bend your right knee and lift your right foot bringing it to the center.
- Place the sole of your right foot on the inner left thigh. You can start right above the knee. As you are more comfortable, you can progress to the point where you cannot bring your leg any higher.

- Press your palms together in front of your chest and raise them above your head. Look straight ahead.

Stay in the Tree Pose from 10 seconds to 20 seconds. Repeat on the other side.

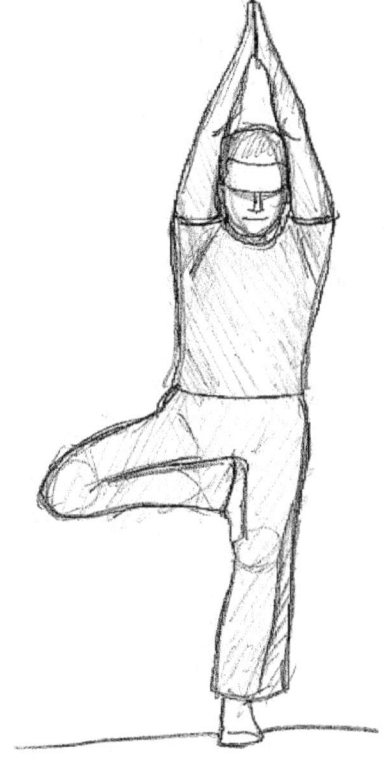

Fig. 137: Tree Pose

Warrior III
Bend forward. Extend your arms in front of you, parallel to the floor. Step your left leg back. Shift your weight to the front leg. Raise your back leg to the balanced position. Try to maintain your body in a straight line, parallel to the floor. This is the Warrior III Pose. Stay in it for 30 seconds.
Repeat on the other side.

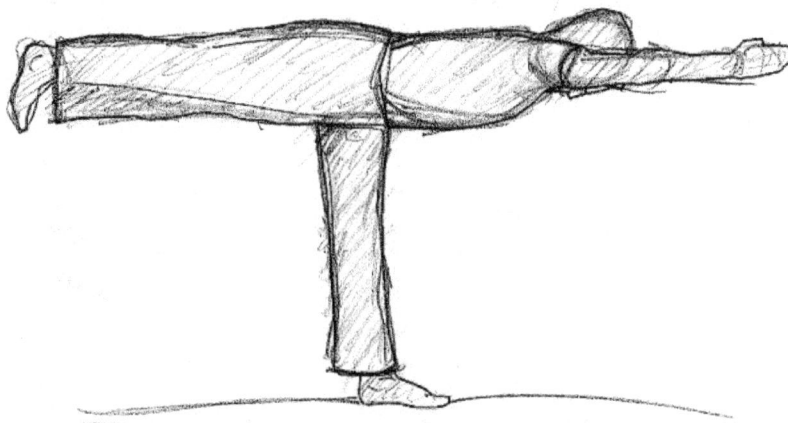

Fig. 138: Warrior III

Plank Pose

Place palms on the floor just outside of the feet. Step right foot back into lunge, lower hips. Step your left leg back into push-up position (top of push-up). The arms should be straight and perpendicular to the floor. Shoulders directly over the wrists, torso parallel to the floor. The feet should be on the balls. Backs of your legs and torso should form a straight line.

This pose strengthens your arms. However, there is a variation of this pose, also called plank, were arms are bent at the elbows (forearms rest on the floor) and it works on abdominal muscles.

Note:

There is a variation of the Plank pose called Dolphin Plank. The only difference is that the arms are bent, and the weight rests on the elbows. This pose is very popular because it strengthens the abdominal muscles.

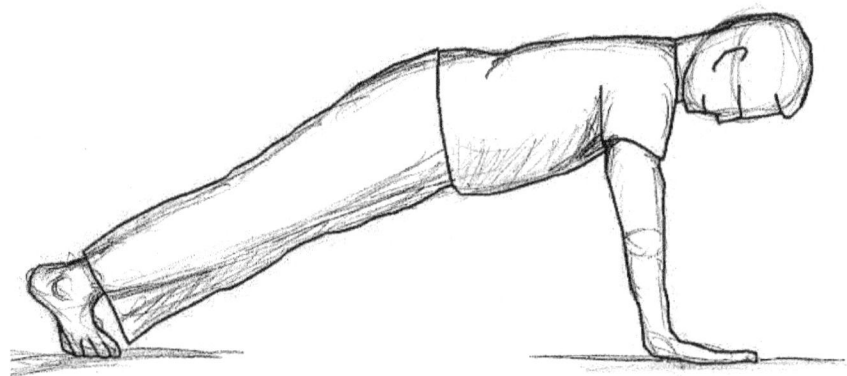

Fig. 139: Plank Pose

Four-Limbed Staff Pose

Exhaling bend elbows and lower body toward floor until it is 4 in above it (lower push-up position). Gaze down. Hold for 10 seconds.

If you lower your body slowly to the floor it maybe better then 2-3 pushups.

Unlike in any other pose, in this pose you will feel that you are using your muscles. You will have control your descent and then hold your body just off the floor for 30 or more seconds. Four-Limbed Staff Pose is one of the positions in the Sun Salutation sequence. You can also practice this pose individually. To come out you can either push up upper body (Cobra Pose) or whole body (Plank Pose).

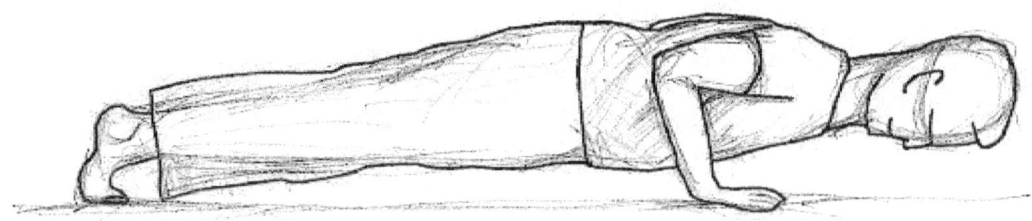

Fig. 140: Four-Limbed Staff Pose

Cobra Pose

Inhaling, roll your feet over the tips of your toes (the feet may also stay on the balls), lower your hips and thighs toward the floor (touch or almost touch the floor), lift your chest on straight arms. Look straight up.

This pose will strengthen your spine, stretch the chest, shoulders, and abdomen, firm the buttocks, and relieve stress and fatigue.

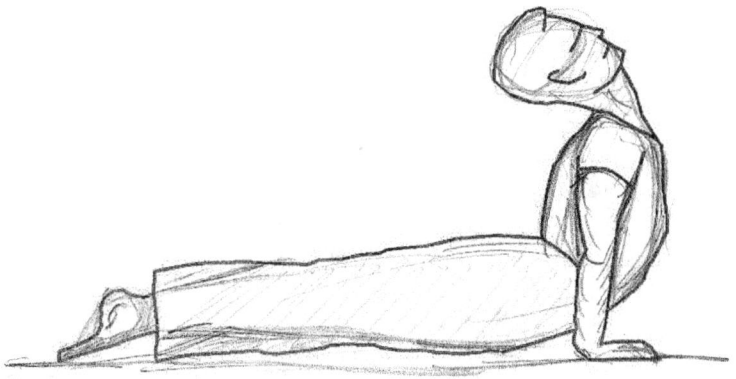

Fig. 141: Cobra Pose

Superman Pose

1. Lie face-down on the floor, feet together, chin on the floor.
2. Stretch the arms in front of you as far as you can.
3. Breathing in, raise the upper torso, arms, and legs. Keep your elbows and knees straight.
4. Hold and continue with long, gentle breaths (in and out). Breathing out, release and relax.

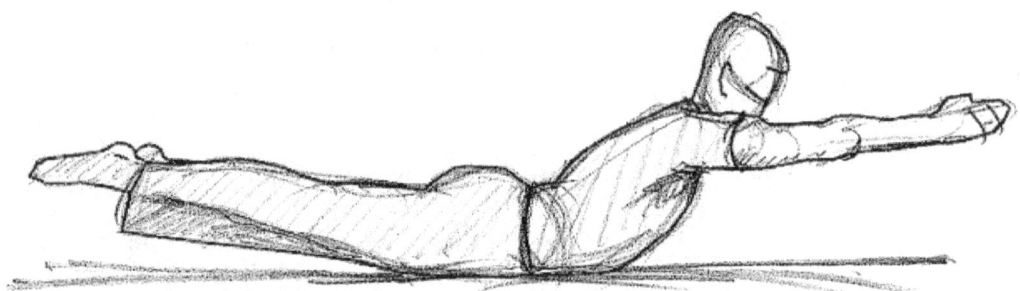

Fig. 142: Superman Pose

Benefits:
Tones the arms and legs. Strengthens abdominal muscles and lower back.

Locust Pose

• Lie on your belly with your arms along the sides of your torso, palms up.
• Rotate your thighs by turning your big toes toward each other. Firm your buttocks.
• Exhale and lift your head, upper torso, arms, and legs away from the floor.
• Raise your arms parallel to the floor and stretch them back through your fingertips.
• Gaze forward or slightly upward.

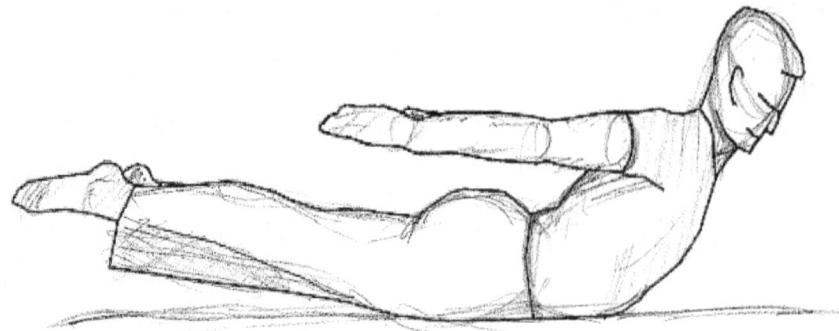

Fig. 143: Locust Pose

Stay in the pose from 10 seconds to 20 seconds, then release with an exhalation. Take a breath and repeat 1 or 2 times.

Bridge Pose
- Lie down on the floor. Arms on the sides.
- Bend your knees and place your feet firmly on the floor as close to your buttocks as possible.
- Lift your hips off the floor. Keep your arms flat on the floor. Your feet and thighs should be parallel, 4 - 6 inches apart. Lift your hips as much as you can. The knees should be directly over the heels. Your spine should arch so you much that only top your shoulder, neck and back of your head touch the floor.

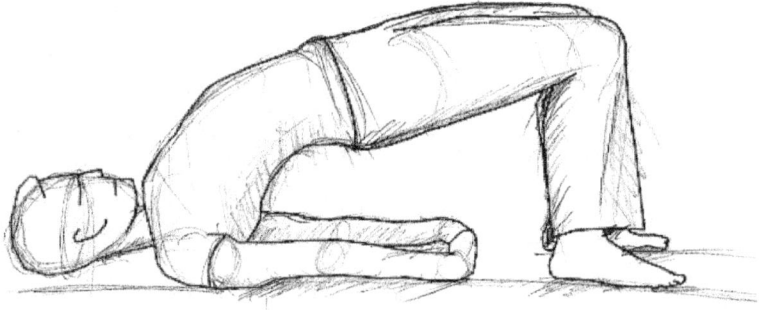

Fig. 144: Bridge Pose

Stay in the Bridge Pose for 10 seconds or little more. When you release from the pose roll the spine down slowly onto the floor.

Half Boat Pose
- Lie supine on the mat.
- Lift your legs 6 inches above the floor.
- Lift your upper body 6 inches above the floor with hands along the body. Hold for 30 seconds. Both legs and upper body are only a half the distance from the floor, hence… Half Boat Pose. Hold it for 10 seconds.

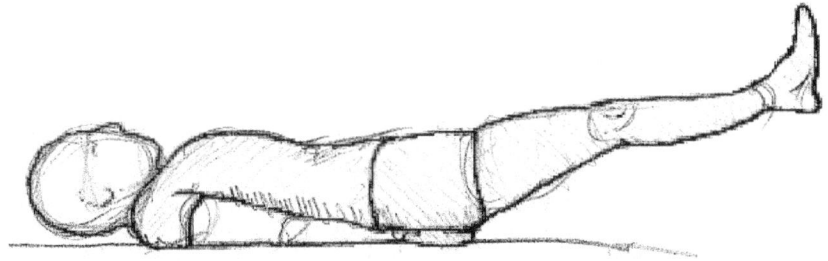

Fig. 145: Half Boat Pose

Full Boat Pose
Sit on the floor with your legs in front of you. Knees can be lightly bent. Lean back slightly and extend your arms in front of you. Lift your legs and straighten them so they are plus/minus 45 degrees from the floor.

If you ever "google" this pose and look at the images the search returns, you will see that there are many ways to get to this pose. Each one is correct. The differences are the result of differences in our bodies and how we accomplish the balance.

Because the balance is not that easy, your pose may look differently every time you try.

Stay in the Full Boat Pose from 10 seconds to 1 minute.

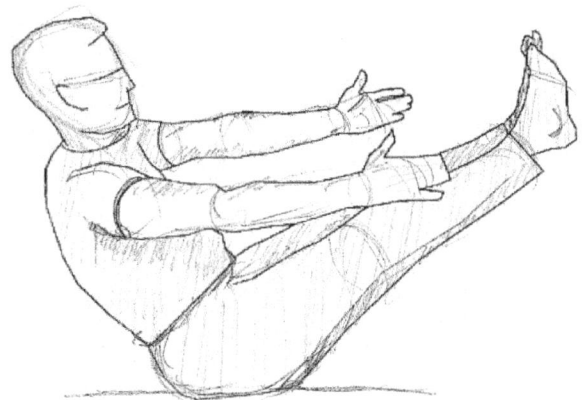

Fig. 146: Full Boat

Head to the Knee:
- Sit with straight legs in front of you.
- Pull the left leg to the center and place the foot sole lightly against the inner thigh of the right leg so the shin is at a right angle to the right leg.
- While holding the left ankle with the left hand grab the right ankle with the other hand. Pull your head to the right knee. Hold for 5-10 seconds.
- Repeat on other side.

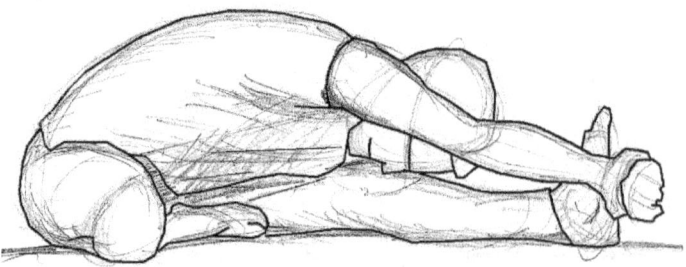

Fig. 147: Head to knee

Spinal Twist:
- Sit with straight legs in front of you.
- Pull the left leg to the center and place the foot under the right leg almost to the buttock.
- Bend the right leg at the knee and place the foot on the floor outside your left thigh. The right knee should point straight up.
- Twist your upper body so that your left shoulder points at the right knee and right shoulder point to the back.
- Place your left hand on the outside thigh of the right leg trying to grab the leg as low as possible.
- The right arm either supports your body. This is the Half Spinal Twist. Stay in it for 5 seconds.
- Repeat on other side.

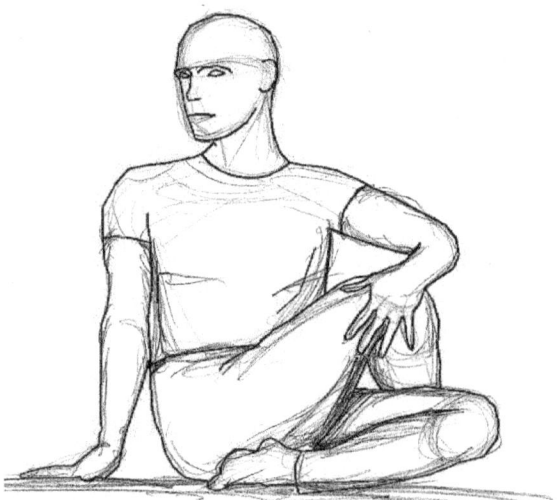

Fig. 148: Spinal Twist

Seated Forward Bend:
- Sit on the floor with your legs straight in front of you.
- Lean forward from the hip joints, not the waist.
- Try to lengthen the front torso into the pose, keeping your head raised.
- Clasp your hands around the ankles and slightly pull into deeper bend.
- Bend the elbows out to the sides.
- Hold for 5 seconds.

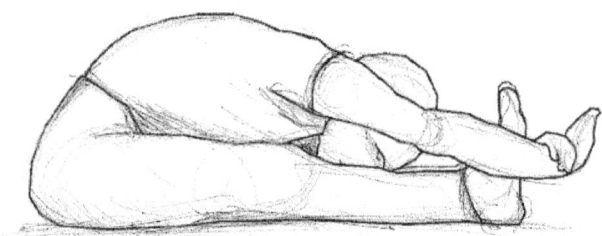

Fig. 149: Forward Bend

Bound Angle Pose

- Sit with your legs out in front of you.
- Exhale, bend your knees and pull your heels toward your center. Put the soles of your feet together.
- Grasp the big toe, or ankle, of each foot. Let your legs open up. Instead of forcing your knees down you can lean forward with your torso. This movement will help open up your hips by gently pushing your knees down.
- Stay in the Angle Pose for 30 seconds.
- Inhale. Extend your legs in front of you.

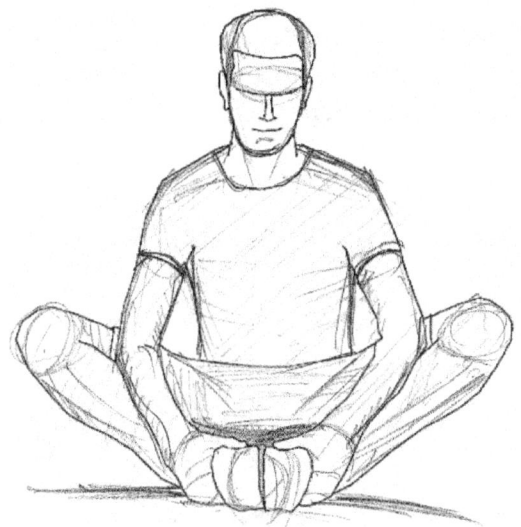

Fig. 150: Bound Angle Pose

Plow Pose

- Lie down on the floor.
- Bring your legs over your head and slowly lower them floor beyond your head.
- Keep your torso perpendicular to the floor and your legs fully extended.
- Press your hands against your back.
- Hold the pose for 10 seconds.
- Start rolling out of the pose.

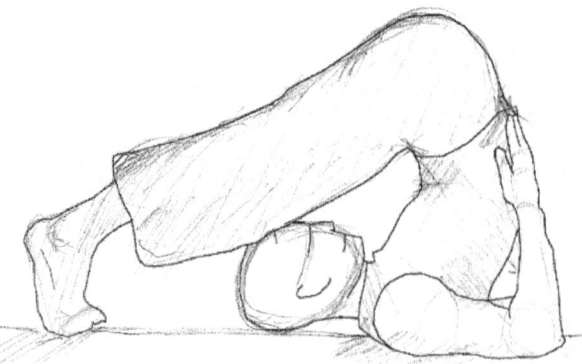

Fig. 151: Plow Pose

Supported Shoulder Stand
- Slowly continue the rolling out motion from previous pose.
- Raise your legs straight up. Lift your lower back up as much as you can (Fig. 57). Keep your bent arms on your lower back locking your upper body in a supported position. Make sure your body is not bent at your hips.
- When your legs are at your highest point make your final pull at your core (or center, or abdominal).
- Stay in the Shoulder Stand Pose for 10 seconds.
- Slowly lower your legs. Then stop supporting your upper body. Slowly bring your legs over your head and lower (unroll) them to the Corpse Pose.

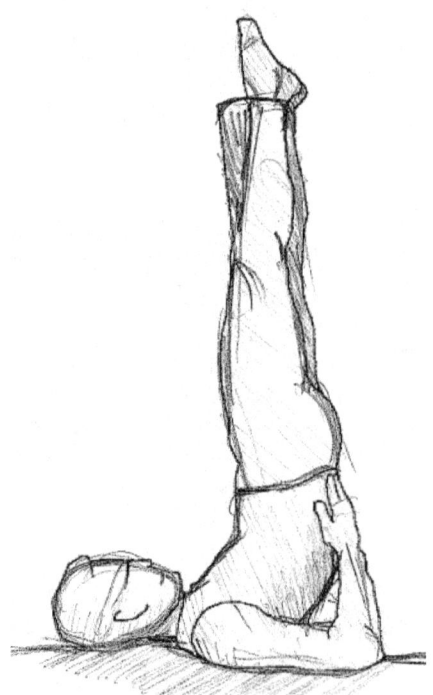

Fig. 152: Shoulder Stand

Rest or Corpse Pose:
- Lie down. Try to get your body into neutral position.
- Extend your arms alongside your body resting backs of the hands on the floor.
- Let shoulder blades rest evenly on the floor.
- Relax all your muscles.
- Stay in this pose 10-20 seconds.

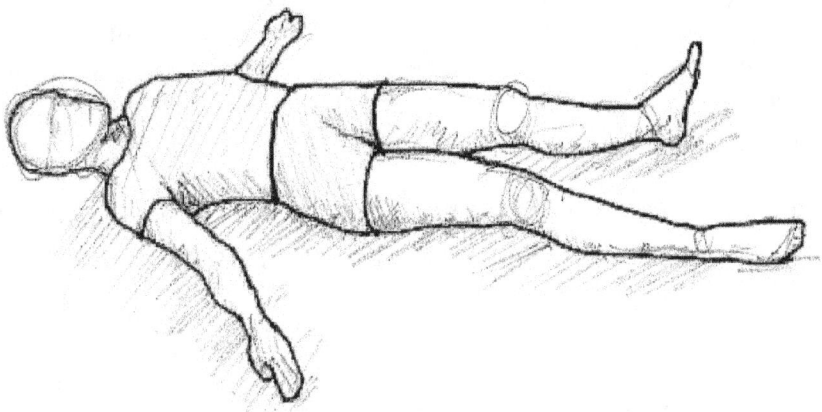

Fig. 153: Corpse Pose

Phase 5 checklist can be found at: http://yoga-connect.blogspot.com/

Office Yoga

Many of us work in the office environment. Usually, we work long hours with very little chances for any physical activity. If you think: "that can't be good", you are absolutely correct. Siting at your desk in front of computer for long hours may result in stress, back pain, repetitive stress injuries, high blood pressure and hearth problems. Just taking a few minutes to do simple yoga exercises at your desk can relieve stress, increase productivity, and most importantly, make you feel better and younger.

Most of the exercises presented are are based on yoga's sitting poses so they should look familiar. The poses are <u>not in any particular order</u>. Do one or two when opportunity arises.

Head Up & Down

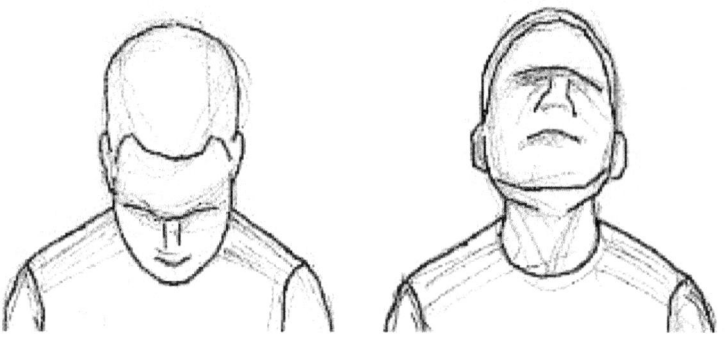

Fig. 154

- Sit on the chair in the neutral pose. Look straight ahead.
- Turn your head up. Look straight up.
- Turn your head down. Look straight down.

Repeat 3 more times.

Head Turns
- Sit up in the neutral pose. Look straight ahead.
- Turn your head 90 degrees to the left. Hold.
- Turn back to look straight ahead. Hold.
- Turn your head 90 degrees to the right. Hold.

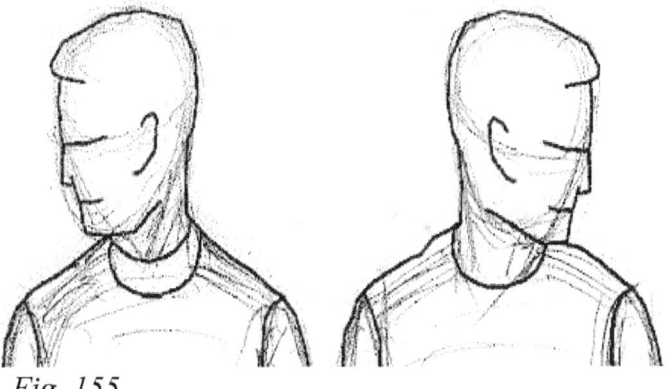

Fig. 155

Repeat 3 more times.

Neck Stretches

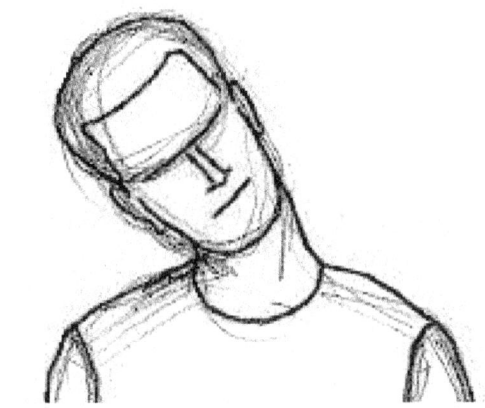

Fig. 156

- With hands resting on your waist, gently lower your chin to relax the back of your neck (the only area that is bent is your neck).
- Hold through 2-3 breaths, return upright to neutral posture.
- Lower your right ear down towards your right shoulder.
- Hold through 2-3 breaths. Relax the left side of your neck.
- Return upright.
- Repeat on the other side.
- Hold through 2-3 breaths. Relax the right side of your neck.

Head rotation
- Sit up in the neutral pose. Look straight ahead.
- Turn your head up. Look straight up.
- Slowly, VERY SLOW, circle your head to the left. Perform a whole circle 4 times.
- Return to the original position. Look straight ahead.
- Slowly, circle your head to the right. Perform a whole circle 4 times.
- Return to the original position.

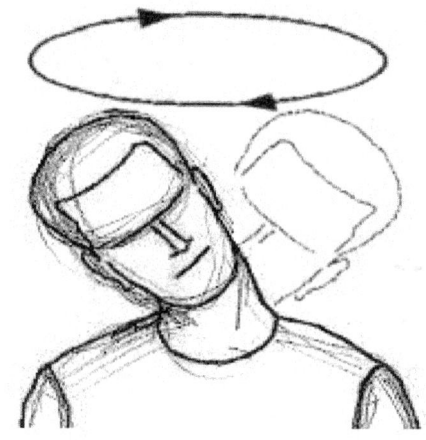

Fig. 157

Repeat two more times.

Side stretch
- Sit straight up in your chair.
- Raise your right hand. Lean to your left while your chest faces front.
- Hold for 2 breaths.
- Come back. Raise your left hand. Lean to your right while your chest faces front.
- Hold for 2 breaths.
- Repeat 2 times.

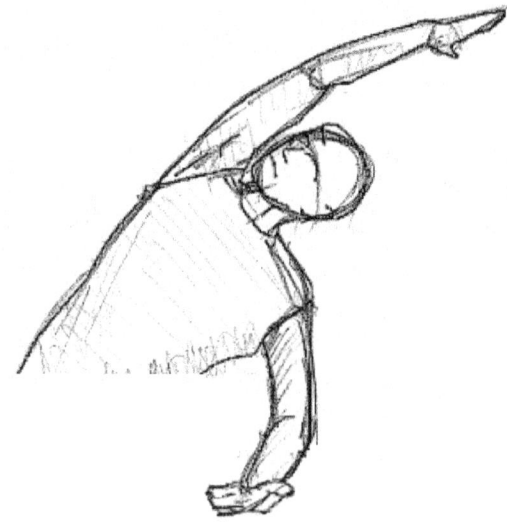

Fig. 158

Overhead Stretch
- Sit straight up in your chair with legs on shoulder width.
- Inhale as you reach up, interlace fingers and turn your palms so they face up.
- Stretch your arms over your head, pull your arms as far to the back as you can.
- Hold for several breaths.

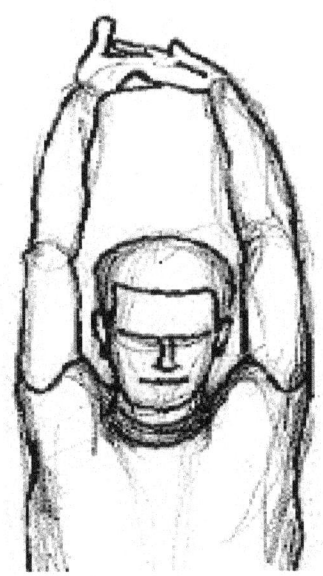

Fig. 159

Downward Dog

- Place yours arms on the desk, shoulder width.
- Lower your head between arms. Arch your back.
- Hold for several breaths.

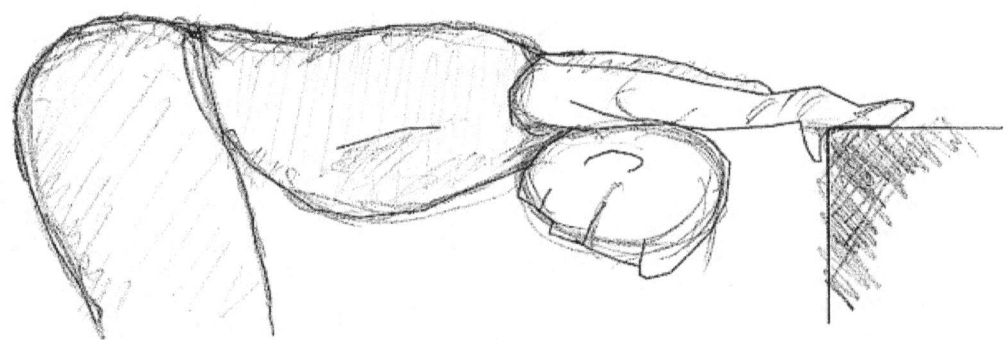

Fig. 160

Wrist Stretch

- Hold up one hand in front of you like you would when saying "stop."
- Grab your fingers with your other hand and pull your fingers back gently to provide a stretch to your wrist.
- Relax your shoulders, and hold through four breaths.
- Repeat on the other hand.

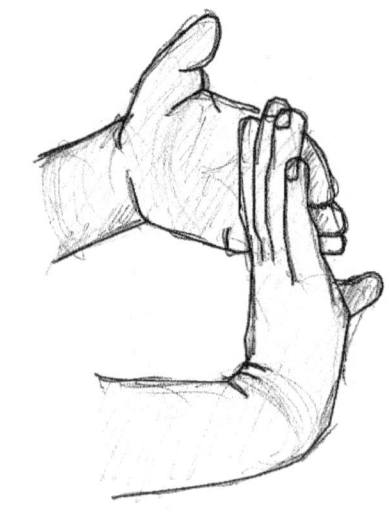

Fig. 161

Shoulder stretch

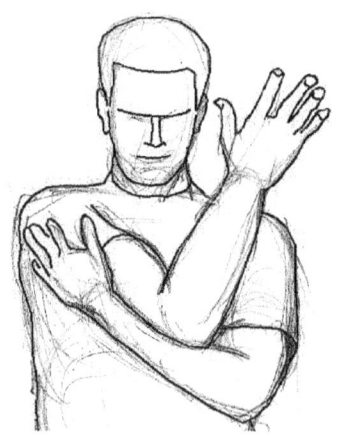

Fig. 162

- Place your right hand on your left shoulder.
- Put your left hand above the elbow of your right arm.
- Press on the elbow so the arm goes beyond left shoulder.
- Hold for 2-3 breaths.
- Repeat on other side.

Abdominal Breathing
- Sit in comfortable pose. Relax your shoulders.
- Inhale. Feel your abdomen expand like a balloon.
- Slowly contract your abdomen by "sucking" in your belly button - exhale.
Repeat 3 more times.

Notes:
If possible, inhale through your nostrils, and exhale through your mouth. Stop the exercise immediately if you feel at all light-headed (proper abdominal breathing should not cause this). When you inhale, try not to lift your shoulders; let the breath "move" into your stomach.

Core Exercises

Exercising your core is important and while yoga poses also work your core it's not always enough. Strong abdominal and back muscles are essential for doing everyday tasks, like lifting a 20-pound toddler and putting away groceries, not to mention preventing an achy back and maintaining good posture at your desk.

The following core exercises are simple but effective. They are meant to be performed in one (1) set each, 5-10 repetitions in each set. Number of repetitions depends on you. If you are short of time perform 5 reps each and it should be enough.

Sit-up/The Roll Up
- Lie on your back on the floor.
- Place your hands at your sides.
- Float your hands up above your head, take a breath and then
- pull yourself up into a seated position for four seconds.
- Breathe out through the mouth. Hold for 2 seconds.
- Breathe in and slowly, roll back down. You should roll back down so slowly that you can feel each vertebra in your back hit the mat one at a time.
- Return to original position.

- Repeat 5 times.

Reverse sit-up
- Lie on your back on the floor.
- Slowly lift your legs up, while breathing in, until they are strait up (90 degrees to the floor).
- Hold for 2 seconds.
- Slowly lower your legs down while breathing out.

- Repeat 5 times.

Sit-up/The Roll Up (no hands)

- Lie on your back on the floor.
- Place your hands at your sides.
- Take a breath and then pull yourself up into a seated position for four seconds.
- Breathe out through the mouth. Hold for 2 seconds.
- Breathe in and slowly, roll back down. You should roll back down so slowly that you can feel each vertebra in your back hit the mat one at a time.
- Return to original position.

- Repeat 5 times.

Criss-Cross

- Lie on your back on the floor.
- Lift (6 inches) your upper-body and legs of the floor.
- Pull both legs to your chest.
- Extend your left leg wihle turning your upper-body so the right elbow touches left knee
- Repeat on other side. Do 10 to 20 twists or crosses at moderate speed.

Final Notes

The program I presented here is similar to the program I followed when I decided that yoga will become part of my life. While I recommend that you practice Yoga at least 3 times a week I practiced every day during my first year. If I didn't have time I would switch to my short schedule that consisted of just Sun Salutations because I thought that with Salutations I will get the best workout in few minutes.

I would like to suggest that after your first year you start experimenting to see what fits your body best. Please visit different Yoga schools and see what they do. Their poses might be different. Their approach might be different then yours. That's OK.

Please sign-up for my on-line program, Yoga Connect, at *http://yoga-connect.blogspot.com/*. I will do my best to present new poses and new routines. I will ask for your thoughts and opinions. We may learn from each other.

Also, please visit my website, *www.fortisyoga.com*, you will like it.

"Live long and prosper" but most importantly, have fun!

Yours,

Kris